How to Heal and Not have the C

FOOD
INFORMATION
FOR ALL PEOPLE

"New Food People," Juicing, Blending, Food Processor People,
Vegan People, Vegetarian People, Cooked Food People,
Animal Milk and Meat People

S HARON J ACOBS

To order additional copies of this book, contact:
Xlibris
1-888-795-4274
www.Xlibris.com
Orders@Xlibris.com

ISBN: 978-1-9845-7915-7 (sc)
ISBN: 978-1-9845-7914-0 (e)

Print information available on the last page

Rev. date: 08/10/2020

Food
Information
for All People

"Fruit, Vegetable, Water, People,"
Juicing, Blending, Food Processor People,
Vegan People,
Vegetarian People,
Cooked Food People,
Animal Milk and Meat People

How to Heal and Not have the Coronavirus

Sharon Jacobs

Sharon Jacobs

Vegetarian- 1980   Vegan- 1998   Juicing- 1999 Fruit, Vegetable, Water - 2011

Ideas

To start having the world of people, eat only garden and farm foods, new from plants and trees, and drink pure water, every day and forever.

To stop the eating of animal's meat, drinking of animal's milk, and eating animal's milk foods, today, permanently, forever.

To stop wearing animal skins of: leather, feathers, fur, and wool. And wear cotton, linen, fleece, velvet, and vinyl, clothes, shoes, and items.

Book Description

Hi, I'm writing to tell you, that I'm a Vegan, Fruit, Vegetable, and Water, Person. And, I was inviting you to be a Vegan, Fruit, Vegetable, and Water, Person also. A New Food People. I eat fruits and vegetables all new, I don't eat the seeds of them, not cooked, and I drink water. I eat only from the plants and trees, of the land, earth, world, and planet, of the universe.

I like to eat all of my foods, of the gardens and farms, new the way that they are made solid, still, quiet, kind, with the soil, rain water, air wind, sunlight, and moonlight, all natural. My favorite fruit is the grapefruit, I like avocados for vegetables. They are nice to eat, all new garden and farm foods. I like it nice like that. And, I planted a garden and farm, in the yard.

If I ate cooked foods, they are vegan, with no animal's meat, or animal's milk, or animal's milk foods, in them.

I don't eat any animal meat of: cow, chicken, egg, turkey, bee honey, pig, fish, shrimp, crab, lobster, oyster, lamb, deer, or other animals. I don't drink or eat any animal dairy milk from cow, or goat, of: milk, cheese, butter, sour cream, cottage cheese, ice cream, chocolate, yogurt, ranch, or whey. I don't wear any animal skins of: leather, feathers, fur, imitation fur, or wool: pants, shirts, skirts, vests, belts, shoes, coats, wallets, purses, sofas, chairs, rugs, pillows, blankets, cars, trucks, motorcycle, or boat seats. I used to, yet not any more. I wear cotton, linen, fleece, velvet, and vinyl, clothes and shoes. I was thinking that this information, might save my life, might save your life, or that might save the life of the animals, and make your life nicer, and make your life, more garden and farm friendly, for our life here on earth.

Now that I know this, and do this, what could I do to make it better? Share that with you. This is a Spiritual way of living, and being on earth for life. And I was thinking, could you do the same, with all of this health information? I know this will be nice for me, for you, for us, and for the world. This book is inspirational about not eating cooked foods, animals, and eating new foods.

About the Writer

Sharon Marie Jacobs was born in Massachusetts. She grew up in Illinois. She wrote the book in Louisiana. She graduated from Utah State University, with a Bachelor in Interior Design. Her hobbies include: writing books, reading, looking at the computer, hiking in the mountains, taking walks in parks of nature, looking at rocks, thinking at home, and doing interior design.

She has been a vegetarian, since age 14, of stopping eating meat and drinking milk. She later became a vegan, eating no meat, and no milk drinks, or milk foods, of all animals, age 32. She is a new food person eating only fruits, vegetables, and water age 45. Being a new food person, is one of the most important things in her life, as she likes this life path. She wrote this book at a nice time in her life, over the years from her experience. The book is about her life experiences, and new foods.

Sharon Jacobs, Vegan, Fruit, Vegetable, Water, Person, in America. Thank You

I have a YouTube video, type in - Sharon Jacobs vegan. Could you watch the video there?

I have a Facebook page - Sharon Jacobs – from Louisiana

This Book is especially for:

Farmers - who plant, water, pick, and sell: fruits, vegetables, and water – all new foods

Food Stores – who have and sell mostly only all new fruits, vegetables, and water

Stores – who have and sell cotton, linen, fleece, velvet, and vinyl fabric clothes, shoes, furniture, cars, and other items

Fruit, Vegetable, Water, People

Vegan People

Vegetarian People

People who ate cooked foods

People who ate animal's meat

People who drank animal's milk

People who hunted, land animals

People who hunted, air animals

People who hunted, ocean animals

People who had a business of animal's, meat food

People who had a business of animal's, milk drinks

People who had a business of animal's, milk foods

People who had a business of restaurants that sell, of animal's meat for food, and animal's milk for drinks

People who had a business of stores, of animal's skins leather, feathers, fur, wool, and animals fabrics, for clothes, shoes, cars, and other items

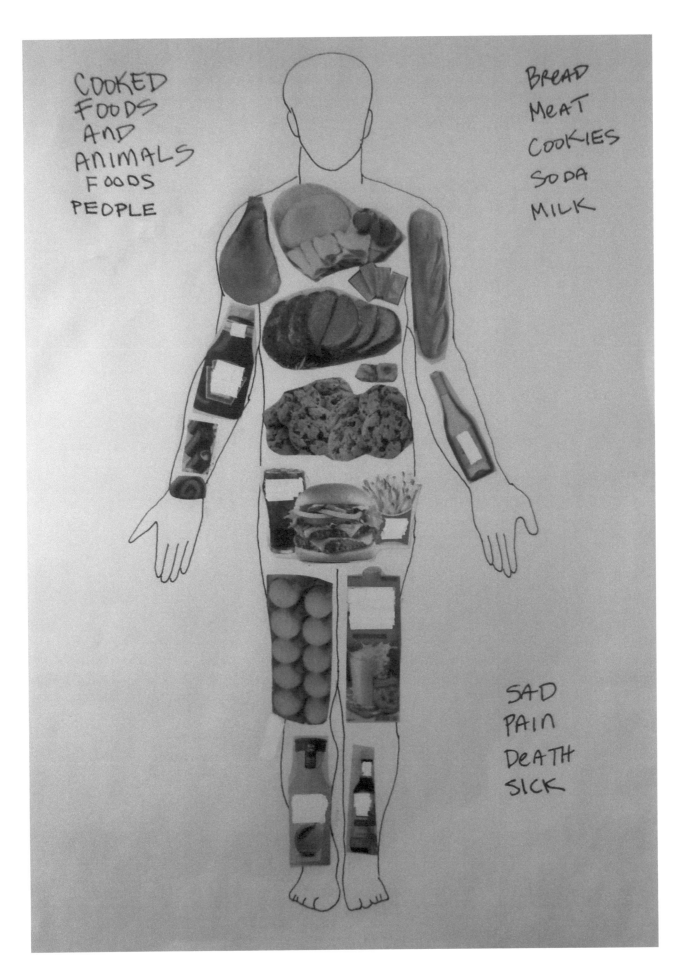

CODKED
FOODS
AND
ANIMALS
FOODS
PEOPLE

BREAD
MEAT
COOKIES
SODA
MILK

SAD
PAIN
DEATH
SICK

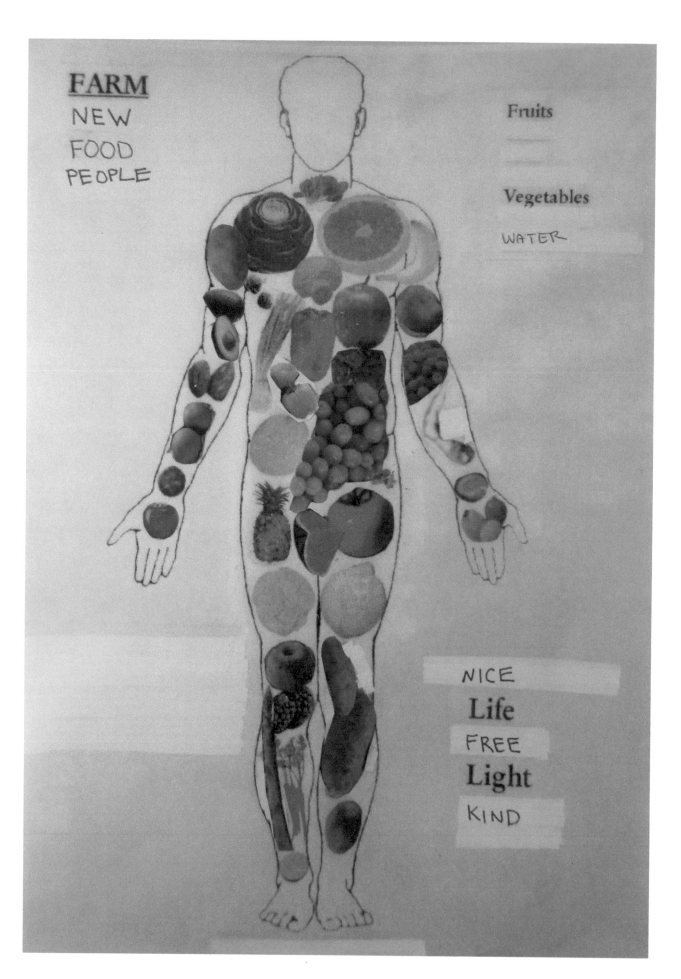

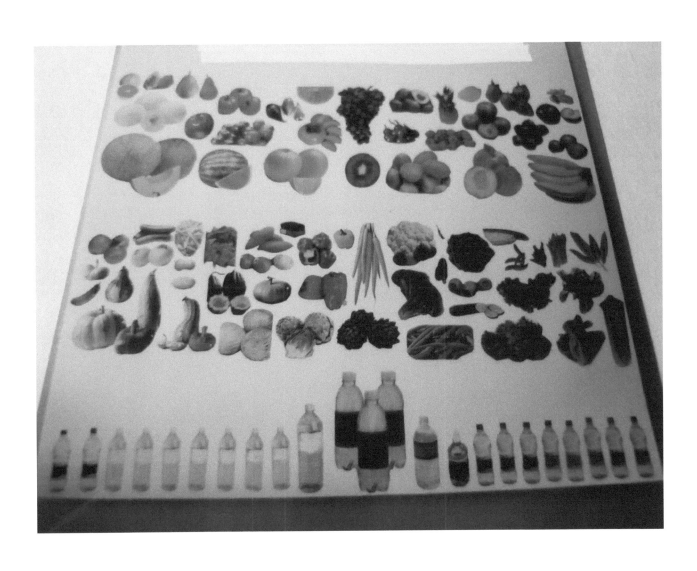

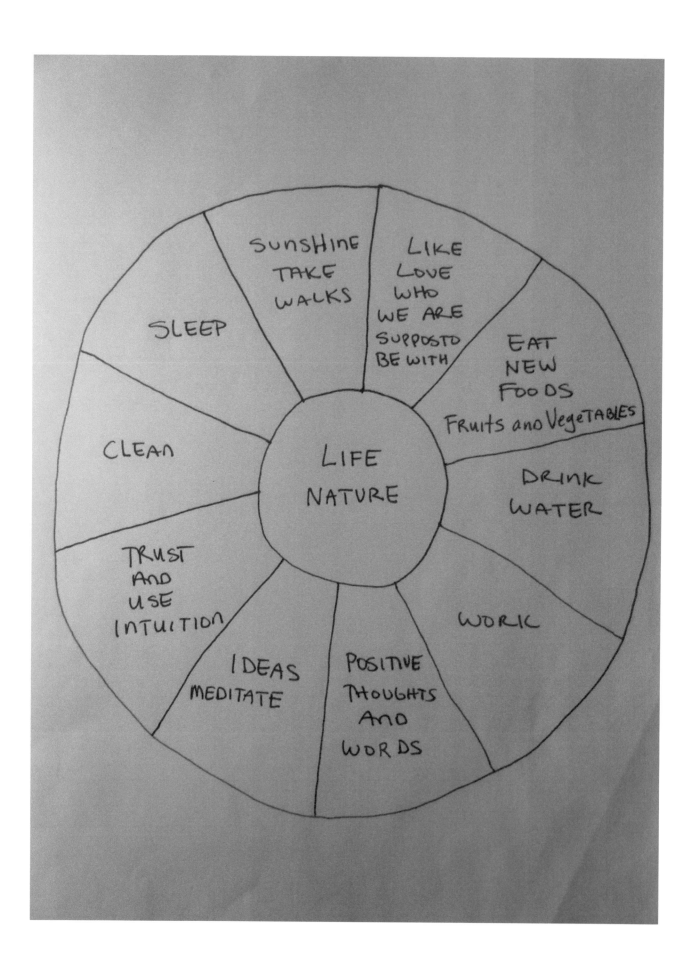

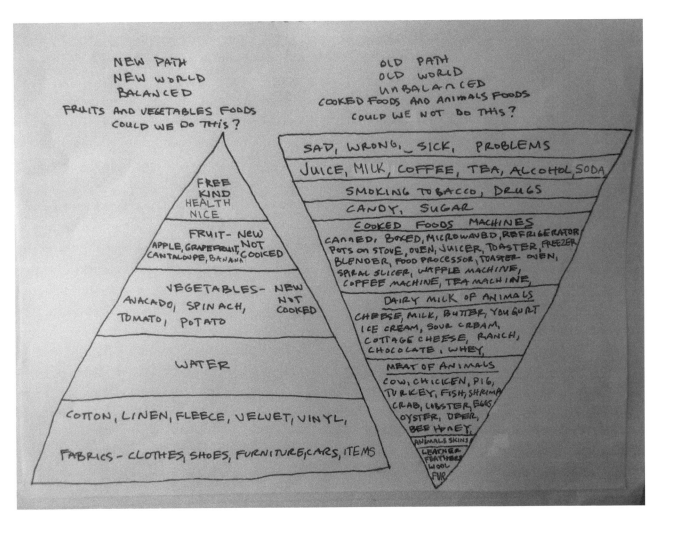

NEW PATH
NEW WORLD
BALANCED
FRUITS AND VEGETABLES FOODS
COULD WE DO THIS?

OLD PATH
OLD WORLD
UNBALANCED
COOKED FOODS AND ANIMALS FOODS
COULD WE NOT DO THIS?

FREE
KIND
HEALTH
NICE

FRUIT- NEW
NOT
APPLE, GRAPEFRUIT, COOKED
CANTALOUPE, BANANA

VEGETABLES- NEW
NOT
ANACADO, SPINACH, COOKED
TOMATO, POTATO

WATER

COTTON, LINEN, FLEECE, VELVET, VINYL,

FABRICS - CLOTHES, SHOES, FURNITURE, CARS, ITEMS

SAD, WRONG, SICK, PROBLEMS

JUICE, MILK, COFFEE, TEA, ALCOHOL, SODA

SMOKING TOBACCO, DRUGS

CANDY, SUGAR

COOKED FOODS MACHINES
CANNED, BOXED, MICROWAVED, REFRIGERATOR,
POTS ON STOVE, OVEN, JUICER, TOASTER, FREEZER,
BLENDER, FOOD PROCESSOR, TOASTER OVEN,
SPIRAL SLICER, WAFFLE MACHINE,
COFFEE MACHINE, TEA MACHINE,

DAIRY MILK OF ANIMALS
CHEESE, MILK, BUTTER, YOGURT
ICE CREAM, SOUR CREAM,
COTTAGE CHEESE, RANCH,
CHOCOLATE, WHEY,

MEAT OF ANIMALS
COW, CHICKEN, PIG,
TURKEY, FISH, SHRIMP
CRAB, LOBSTER, EGGS,
OYSTER, DEER,
BEE HONEY,
ANIMALS SKINS
LEATHER
FEATHER
WOOL
FUR

7

Man and Woman, Nature, and Food

In the start of the world, a time on earth, where the first people, had the idea, and nice plan, to have only man and woman, him and her, who their supposto be with, nature, food, a metal house, and metal and wood furniture to live with. They eat only from fruits, vegetables, all new from plants and trees, from the gardens and farms, not cooked, and they drink water only.

They wore clothes made from plants, of the land of cotton, linen, fleece, velvet, and vinyl clothes and shoes. They stay at home most of the day, and night in their house, yet they take walks in nature near the house and at parks. They talk to each other. They planted a garden and farm, and planted fruit trees, nut trees, and vegetable plants on the land. They are nice and live kind on the earth, on this planet, in the universe. They are leaders and examples, of what to do in life. They are a new food people. They made the perfect science: nature, mountains, lakes, streams, trees, grass, rocks, flowers, fruits and vegetables with water. They are doctors of fruits, vegetables, and water, and cotton, linen, fleece, velvet, and vinyl clothes and shoes, and other items.

They do service work in the home, garden, and farm. A garden and farm is where people plant trees, and plants, that grow food for them to eat, at home in their back yard, or at the farm. They plant vegetable and fruit plants, that grow food for them to eat. They plant trees that grow food fruit and almonds to eat. They pick their food from the garden and farms, and eat their foods new. They don't eat old food. They keep their foods on the counters, at nature's temperature, in the kitchen of the house.

They don't use a refrigerator, pots on the stove, oven, microwave, Juicer, food processor, blender, coffee machine, tea machine, toaster, toaster oven, waffle machine, sandwich machine, dehydrator, crock pot, can opener, or juice press. The first people didn't eat dead animals bodies flesh, red blood, and white blood fat, called meat. They didn't drink from live animal's utters, of white blood fluids, called milk. They didn't wear dead animals bodies skins, with the fur or hair removed from that, called leather, feathers, fur, imitation fur, or wool, for clothes, and shoes. They didn't use dead animal's skins called leather on: sofas, chairs, rugs, car seats, truck seats, motorcycle seats, or other items.

We too should live life like that, not using animals, and not eating animal's meats, or drinking animal's milks, for all of our lifes, because farm foods are of the land, of plants and trees, for we. That is powerful and truthful. Imagine a world like that, all natural, of nature of plants and trees foods, clothes, and items, they are here for we. They know the path we should take and do, to eat healthy foods and drink healthy water, wear healthy clothes and shoes, and use healthy items of furniture, and cars.

Eating only garden and farm foods, of plant and tree foods, of fruits and vegetables, and drink water, from nature, the land, world, earth, planet, and universe, for we is healthy, protection, safe, quality, connection, independent, clarity, success, necessary, truth, important, excellent, pure, knowledge, special, achievement, complete, value, support, nutrition, kind, fine, happy, security, power, value, right, fulfillment, fitness, royal, better, supreme, solutions, original, friendly, care, mature, real, calm, commitment, solid, light, awesome, perfect, energy, quality, truthful, unique, hope, vision, balance, new, elegant, clean, high, worthy, peaceful, freshness, necessary, intelligent, positive, nature, life, centered, commitment, beautiful, favorite, nice, creation, alive, natural, inspirational, spiritual, love, like, and freedom.

Imagine a world, of all people all like this, eating and drinking, wearing, and using, only garden and farm new foods, and garden and farm material fabric for clothes, shoes, and items. Could we do this now, today, yesterday, tomorrow, and forever as new food people?

I think that all homes, restaurants, school, businesses, and stores should be like that, and only have or sell, garden and farm foods, and new fruits and vegetables of foods to the people, and use cotton, linen, fleece, velvet, and vinyl clothe, shoes, and items like they did in the start of the world. We should not eat animal's bodies or milk foods, we should not be in those places that serve animals to eat. Not eat animal's meat, and not drink animal milk, should not be sold, to protect the animals, and to help us eat, the path we should be eating new, to drink what we should be drinking water only, and wear what we should be wearing cotton clothes and vinyl and fabric shoes, not animals skins leather, clothes and shoes.

All places of business, and homes, should be only serving, food of garden and farm fruit and vegetables, for we to eat, and all of we, that would be better. And the world, would be a better place. More peaceful, quiet, kind, and friendly. Let's have a new tradition and life, on this world of people, on earth of the universe.

The world, used to be like that, a long time ago. Only garden and farm food was in homes, and sold in stores. And the world, was a better place a long time ago, since it was mostly, all garden and farm foods, that were eaten, in the start of creation, and for a while.

This is the kind of world, that I imagine to live in, all living new foods. No dead foods, of animal foods. Only living garden and farm new foods. We could build our body from fruits and vegetables, from plants and trees, of the land and earth, instead of building our body with dead animal's meat bodies and alive animal's milks foods and drinks. We could have a city, and nation, of living life and light, with new foods, fruits, vegetables and water. We can start our own life over, eating new foods at home individually, as a person, even if we are alone, or together as a couple or family? Or we can start a farm at our own home, in the backyard by yourself, or with your husband or wife, and family? And continue your garden, year round at home, and in our city in the world, on earth, of our planet.

Yet, somewhere along the line of people, they began change the original plan, of new fruits and new vegetables. They began to cook the foods of fruits and vegetables, they ate animals, and wore animal's skins of leather, feathers, fur, and wool. Could this be stopped? We must forgive ourselves and forgive them. And start to be back at the start of the world, of how they originally ate, drank, dressed, and made items for use, in the world for our lifes.

We can talk to other people, about what we do of eating only fruits, vegetables with out the seeds and drink water, to inspire them, and teach them, a better way of life. This needs to be done more. We should teach this in our families, schools, work business, citys, and countries of the world. We have to find out, on our own, with our husband or wife, or through a few select people that we meet.

If I could change our world of people, from eating animals, drinking animals, wearing animals, and using animals, I would. I would change our world of eating dead animal foods, and drinking alive animal's milk, to a world of only eating life fruits and vegetables foods only. Could we have a world, of eating only garden and farm foods, new fruits, and new vegetables, and wearing plant material fabric for clothes, shoes, and items? Yes.

Now is the time to prepare. Now is the time to visit the start of the world, when it was nicer and more free. We need a world that is pure and clean, made of nature's earth foods, and nature's items. Not animal foods, animal drinks, animal leather, feathers, fur, imitation fur, and wool clothes, animal leather shoes, animal leather cars and animal leather trucks, or animal items made by man. We must live as they did in the past, in the start of the world, of what was created, plants and trees foods, and materials of fabric for us to eat, drink, and wear. And we must do this now today, yesterday, tomorrow, and forever as a people, in our countries and citys, at home and in the work place.

We have a problem with the world, because people ate the animals, drank the animals, wore the animals, and used the animals for items, so we must fix those problems today and tomorrow.

We have a solution, and that is to first start with our self. I'll start with me. Then, I will help others. I have to live in the now of today, with the world, with our stores, from gardens and farms on the land, of this earth and planet, and we all should be eating and drinking from that. Nature is the solution to eat, drink, wear, and use only garden foods, and farm plant clothes and items. This is nice for our mind, body, and spirit. This is power for our lives to start where we are at, and make a new life, clean and free, with nature's land foods, from plants and trees. Not cooked with no oxygen air, or water in them, or animal foods. Earth foods are made from water, and have water in them.

We must think about this, and remember this, and do this, so we can have a new world, all plant and tree based. Not animals based. It's time for a new place at home, at the stores, and at work, to have, a free world of a healthier path, and I have that with me. So, how about you? How about we? How about the world?

Coronavirus

We are all at home, like being back in the start of time, where the first people stayed in their homes, and had a garden and farmed their own foods in the yard, ate only fruits and vegetables new, from the land and earth, and they took walks, and didn't have extra activities.

And then something happened, the people began to cook their foods, and capture animals and eat them. That is the Coronavirus.

The fact is that the Coronavirus is caused by eating animal's meat flesh bodies, and drinking animal's milk fluids from the animals utters, and wearing animal's skins leather, feathers, fur, and wool. An animal has a head, body, arms, legs, tail from its spine, and fur or hair all over its body. They were captured by people, and cut up to eat, or milked the animal to drink. The animal's bodies flesh is called meat, that they ate. And the animal's bodies white blood fluids is called milk, that they drank. They have drank alive cow fluids milk, and eaten dead cow bodies flesh meat red blood. That is what has caused the Coronavirus. This virus has been happening for centuries, ever since people milked an animal and drank their milk, and captured an animal, and ate their meat. They were sick from doing that, eating an animal and drinking an animal. And so has everyone else who did the same. Sickness is a virus, no matter what the sickness is. And sickness is caused by eating animal's meat, and drinking animal's milk.

The Coronavirus was started from the animals using the bathroom on the land, and not cleaning it up. They leave it there. They can't clean it up. We have to clean it up for them. And the animals have to walk around where they went to the bathroom, sit by it, eat the grass by it, and the bathroom they use gets on them, and in them, and the animals have the Coronavirus first. If we eat animal's meat or drink animal's milk, we will be sick from the meat and milk of animals, and have the Coronavirus. How to stop the Coronavirus is stop eating animals meats, and stop drinking animals milk, and start eating only fruits, and vegetables and water, that will heal the virus from we, in our world.

The only time I was sick was when I was a child, because I ate meat or drank milk of animals. I didn't like being sick, so I stopped eating animals meat, and I stopped drinking animals milk. When I stopped doing that, I wasn't sick anymore. I had a virus when I was a child from eating animals. I was allergic to animals in my body, I just didn't know it. It took me years to learn, what different kinds of meat were animals. And, I felt better eating fruits and vegetables, and drinking water, all fresh, uncooked, because l feel healthy, and I didn't get sick anymore. I don't get sick now for years.

Anyone can be healed and get better from the Coronavirus, simply by stop eating animal meat, and stop drinking milk of animals. All they have to do is eat fresh fruits and vegetables, and drink water, and the virus will leave their body. It has to. The garden and farm foods of plants and trees, will heal your mind, body, and spirit in your life.

The virus started with the hunters who capture the animals alive or dead. The virus started with the business of animals, who take the animals into the buildings, death them, and cut up the animals for food. The virus started with stores that purchase animal's meat and animal's dairy milk, to sell to people to eat and drink. The virus started when restaurants served dead animal meat to eat, and alive animal milk to drink. The virus started when you bought the animal's meat, and animal's milk drink and foods, and ate and drank them.

The Coronavirus ends when you stop purchasing animals meat and milk, and start only purchasing fruits and vegetables, and purchasing water. The virus stops when stores stop selling animals clothes, shoes, and items to the people. The virus stops when restaurants stop serving animals to eat, and serve only fruits, vegetables, with water to drink to the people. The virus stops when the hunters and business of animals stop deathing them and cutting up animals. The virus stops when the hunters stop capturing the animals of the land, air, and ocean and let them live on the land free, away from people.

Farmers don't have the Coronavirus, they have health and life foods, of plants and trees for the people of the world, to eat and drink for we individually, or as a couple, or as a family.

The hospitals are filled with people who are sick, from some kind of sickness, virus, or disease, and they don't know why. It is because people ate animal's bodies meats red blood, and white blood fat, on the meat, or drank animal's milk white blood fluids, and too much cooked foods. Doctors and nurses should inform people, to eat only fruits and vegetables, and drink only water, in their eating and drinking habits, to heal their sicknesses, virus and diseases to be well, to be better, and to be healthier in their life.

I am a vegan, new food person, eating only fruits and vegetables, and drink water some of my life. I am healthy. I have been around people in many cities, who eat animal's meat, and drink animals milk drinks and foods, and I have never caught the virus from people, only from the animals. The animals that were being cooked, on the oven or in the stoves, microwaves, and pots, has steam that is in the air, and the people breathe that, if they are near it, and can get sick. The virus sickness is in the animals, that have been eaten and drank.

We as a individual person, house, or apartment, family, and people, city, country, and world, could we stop eating animals, could we stop drinking animals, and also could we stop wearing animal's leather, feathers, fur, and wool, and stop using animals for clothes, shoes, accessories, furniture covers on sofas, chair, rugs, cars, trucks, motorcycles seats, animal wall mounted plaques, and other items? If we want to heal as a home, city, nation, world, planet and earth, we must do this now today, and every day in the future.

Finally, the world of people in countries, cities, stores, restaurants, and homes are in a stay at home order, from too much excessive shopping and buying, eating and drinking, and doing other extra activities. Now we have time to sit at home, and think about what we have done, to our selves, and to this world of eating animals, and drinking animals, and wearing animals, and using animals for items. We should be throwing away all animals items, that we have in our homes, apartments, and businesses of work. We should be putting new foods in our homes on our tables, counters, refrigerators, and cupboards, stores and work places, of fruits, vegetables, and drink water. And we should be thinking more about new foods, from the farms, of farmers.

While you are at home start to plant a garden in the yard, and grow your own food, plant trees of grapefruit, oranges, apples, pears, cantaloupes, tomatos, avocados, potatos, spinach, and almonds, and pick your own fruits. Plant in the ground, plants of and pick your own vegetables. Plant trees and pick fruits and almonds. Could we stop purchasing animal's meat and animal's milk, and purchase only fruits, vegetables, and drink water, for your home? And this will heal you, heal your family, and heal the homes, citys, countries, nations, and world. This is an experience of being at home, and not driving out so much doing extra activities. We should stay home more and talk to each other. So could we take a walk in your front yard, in front of the house, in nature or walk around the block or at a park, and talk to one another. Sit in the silence, in the quiet, and think about what a new life we could have, as a new individual, family, city, country, and world, of only eating fruits and vegetables, and water.

I've been working on this book for years, and right after I finished writing my book, within a few weeks, the Coronavirus happened. Remember this virus has been happening for thousands of years, based on results of people being sick. Our world is healthy with people who eat only fruits and vegetables, and drink water, and wear clothes made from plants. The world is sick right now with a virus of how they eat, drink, wear, use, and behave, that is animals based. We must only eat from plants and trees, and wear plant fabrics, and do plants activities of being still, kind, and quiet more. The world has a problem and it's my problem too. The world has a solution and its garden and farm foods only. You don't get sick from eating fruits, vegetables, and water, you get better, and you get healthier.

This book will explain my life's experiences of stopping eating animals, drinking animals, and wearing animals, and inform you   vegan, and a new food person, eating only fruits, vegetables and drinking water, all day, every day forever.

My Food Life about Foods and Animals

Animals milk and meat, Vegetarian, Vegan, and Fruit, Vegetable, Water, Person

Sharon Jacobs

Born and grew up eating animals

I have been a vegetarian – stopped eating cow meat, and cow milk - since 1980, age 14

I have been a vegan – stopped eating all animal meat, all animal milk products, and wearing leather - since 1998, age 32

I have been a vegan and juicing person – start eating all fresh fruits, vegetables, nuts, wheat, and rice - since 1999, age 33

I have been a new food person eating fruits and vegetables and water – 2011 age 45

I have been practicing, not eating animals for 40 years, and eating mostly, garden and farm foods, from plants and trees, of the land and earth. I'm now 54

I went from eating animal's meat, drinking animal milk items, and wearing animal clothes, and being sick, to being healed by being a vegetarian, vegan, to new food person, who eats only, garden and farm foods, of plants and trees, of the land, and wearing cotton and linen clothes and fabric and vinyl shoes.

Pig Meat

The first animal meat, I learned to not eat.

I went to high school for the first time, and I was standing in the foyer, when a boy started a conversation with me. He said, "Do you know what's in a hot dog?"

He seemed to be sad, as if he just found out, and had to tell someone.

I said, "No, what?"

And he said, "A pig."

I felt sad, it seemed to get dark. I didn't know that a hot dog, was made up of a pig into food. I was sad at that realization, that a pig was in food. It didn't seem right to me. It thought it was wrong and sad, that a pig was in a hot dog.

I went home that day after school, and I saw that my mom was serving me a hot dog for dinner. I stood in the kitchen and stared at the table, with the food on it.

I thought, "I have a decision to make." Right there, in the kitchen I decided that I was not eating the hot dog, and I never eat them. I only ate the bun with the tomato, lettuce, and mustard. And I never ate pig in any form, not pork chops, not ribs, sausage, and not bacon. And I felt nice about that decision.

I was 14 years old, when I made that decision, to not ever eat pig, from what that boy taught me, in high school my first week there. What he told me about the pig, and the hot dog, I remember to this day. What he told me, changed my life, and I have not eaten a pig to this day. What I learned from that boy, in high school, my first week in ninth grade, I will always remember that. What that boy, taught me was some of the most important information, that I learned in high school. I learned to not eat animals. He taught me that in school. My family didn't even teach me that. Fortunately, I learned from a friend.

I have remained a vegetarian from eating pigs for 40 years, until I am 54 years old, and have felt right about that decision. What he taught me affected me, now for 40 years, and I plan to not eat animals for the rest of my life. I am happy he taught me. I was very lucky to have learned that. I was informed by him, I'm happy, he told me, because it changed my eating habits, for all of my life.

A pig is short and walks on the ground. It has a head, body, arms, legs, and a tail out of its spine. It's usually pink in skin color. It has no hair on its body. People death the pig, and cut it up, to sell to eat called: bacon, ribs, hot dog, bolony, and ham. That is all from the pigs back part of the body. They throw the rest of the pig away of its head, arms, legs, tail, and organs.

Could you not eat animal pig meat?

Could you look at the computer or phone internet search, and type or say, picture of a pig, to see what a pig looks like? To see where pig meat is from of the pig of: bacon, sausage, ribs, bolony, hot dog, and ham.

Cow Meat

One day, I was in my room, in much pain in my stomach. I was bent over, and I had to hold my stomach, because it was hurting so much, in pain for an hour. As I was in that pain I thought, "What did I eat today? Then I thought that, "I ate cow meat." So I said, "What if I stop eating cow meat, maybe my stomach won't hurt."

I thought that my stomach hurt so much, from what I had eaten, and it made since to me to stop eating cow meat, to stop the pain. After that painful time, and awareness, I never ate cow meat again. It was just too much pain, for a 14 year old girl, to experience, and I didn't want to feel that pain again in my body ever.

After I had made the decision, to never eat cow meat again, our family was eating dinner. Meat was served, and I didn't eat it. I didn't have meat on my plate. Then my family noticed, that I didn't have meat on my plate, and said to me, "You need to eat meat." And I said to them, "I can't, it makes me sick."

Then the next day, my family said the same thing to me again, as they noticed, I wasn't eating meat. They said, "You need to eat meat." And I said to them "It hurts my stomach." After I told them that eating meat, made me sick, they stopped saying that to me.

I had to do what I needed to do. I didn't eat cow meat again, and my stomach didn't hurt, like it used to hurt. I was used to being sick from eating meat, and I didn't know that I was so sick, from eating the animal meat, until later in life, when I learned that meat is animals.

So after making the decision to stop eating cow meat, my stomach never ever hurt like that much again. It was worth it for me, to stop eating cow meat, to have no pain. I felt better and happier.

A cow is tall and has a head, big body, arms, legs, and tail out from its spine to cover it. They are usually white, black or brown in color. The cow walks on the ground and eats grass. The people death the cow, cut it up, and sell the back part of the cow for food called: meat, steak, beef, meatloaf and others. They only use the back part of the cow for food and throw the rest of the cow away of its head, organs, arms, legs, and tail.

They use the skin of the cow to make leather. They remove the fur or hair, from the skin leather to make items from it such as leather coats, leather vests, leather pants, leather skirts, leather shirts, leather belts, leather wallets, leather purses, leather hats, leather car seats, leather truck seats, leather motorcycle seats, leather sofas, leather chairs, leather rugs, and other leather items. And leather is animal's skins from the cow's body of its sides and back.

Could you not eat animal cow meat? Could you not wear animal cow leather clothes and shoes? Could you not use cow leather items? Wallets and purses. Could you not sit on animal cow leather sofas, chairs, cars, and trucks?

Could you look at the computer, or on your phone internet search, and type or say, picture of a cow? To see what a cow looks like. And to see where meat, beef, steak, and leather is from on the cow?

Cow Milk

Another day I noticed a smaller pain in my stomach. It was a milder pain, than the pain from the meat. I realized that the lesser pain, was from drinking the cow milk. So, I stopped drinking it, and the pain stopped in my stomach. The pain went away, and I learned that I was lactose intolerant. I couldn't drink milk.

Later in life I found a milk substitute, soy. I began to drink soy milk, I knew it was better for me to drink, than cow milk. And then I found rice milk, and that felt better to drink. I also found that someone made coconut milk so I drank that. And someone also made almond milk. So there are a lot of milk substitutes. I didn't have to drink animal cow dairy milk, when there are other milks, from the garden and farms of the trees, of foods from the earth and land.

And then later, I had a realization from the almond milk that someone had made, in the containers, at the stores is processed, and maybe cooked. So, I thought that I should make my own almond milk. I bought some almonds. I put about a hand full of almonds in the blender, with 2 cups of water and blended the almonds. It made fresh almond milk. It was a white milk consistency, yet thinner. And it tasted nice and new.

And sesame seeds milk makes white milk too. 2 tablespoons of sesame seeds with 2 cups of water blended is very healthy milk to drink. I also tried other nuts to make milk. The nut milk is better for you and fresh, if you make it yourself. Instead of drinking cow milk, it is better for you to drink natural nut milk from the earth, in its natural state, grown from the land of the trees.

Yet, it's nice to drink water though, and not drink milk from nuts or animals.

Cow milk is from the animal female cow. They put a milking machine, that is silver, on the cow's body parts, in the back of the cow, underneath the cow's body, to pump the cow's body from their utters, for milk to be out of the cow, to sell to drink. The milk from the cow is white blood fluids. Cows drink water, and the water in the cow's body, turns to white blood fluids, it's not for people to drink from. We should drink water only, and not drink milk from a cow's body. It hurts them and they don't like being pumped for milk. They want to be left alone and not have that done to them.

Could you not drink animal cow's milk from their body? Let's drink water instead. It's better for we.

Could you look at the picture of a cow on the internet search on your computer or phone to see where the milk is from on a cow?

Vegetarian

After stopping eating pig meat, cow meat, and cow milk for a few years, I learned that I was a vegetarian. That is what it is called when you don't eat some type of meat or dairy milk. So, I worked on not eating those animal meats, and animal milks, on a daily basis. I watched what I ate. I ate mostly salads, vegetables, and fruit. I was the only one, in my family who practiced being a vegetarian. And I didn't know anyone else who ate vegetarian, it was just me alone doing that.

Someone told me first about the animals, and I made a decision that I didn't want to eat them. Then I learned on my own, when I was sick, from eating other meats and milk, so I stopped eating those meats, and I stopped drinking that milk that was animal based.

I learned that it is important, to pay attention to my body, and if it hurts, then something that I ate is wrong and sad. If my body feels sick from eating something, then I need to stop eating that. If eating food that makes me be sick, there is something wrong and sad with it, and I should stop eating it. And animals are not food. Animals are animals. Animals should not be cut up and called meat or milk. And I shouldn't eat them. I feel nicest eating fruits and vegetable, and I feel healthy eating earth foods.

Turkey Meat

I think I ate turkey once.

I was sitting at the table with my family, for Thanksgiving, and I thought, "Thanksgiving is only once a year. So, I could stop eating turkey meat." And I stopped eating turkey right there at the table. And I only ate all of the vegetables.

At Thanksgiving dinner my family asked me, "Why are you not eating Turkey?" I told them that I didn't eat meat. They didn't say anything to me about it. I was happy I made that decision to not eat turkey meat any more. And I haven't eaten any turkey since then.

A turkey is a bird that is supposto fly in the air, yet it can't because it's too big. It walks on the ground. It has a head, body, wings, feet, and a tail. It has black feathers all over its body. They eat all of the body of wings, chest, thighs, and legs, not the head or feet.

Could you look on your phone or computer on the internet search for picture of a turkey to see what they look like?

Chicken Meat

I remember eating my last chicken sandwich, from a food restaurant, as I drove away with my sandwich, I knew that it was the last chicken sandwich, that I would eat. Because I didn't eat pig meat, or cow meat, now I was not going to eat chicken meat.

And then after that, I read in a book, that chicken was some of the most difficult meats, for the body to digest. So, when I read that, I made sure that I stopped eating chicken, that instant. I read that book in 1998, and I still haven't eaten chicken, since reading why I shouldn't eat chicken. I think I had the thought that chicken, was healthier than cow meat, or pig meat, yet that wasn't true. No animal bodies meat is healthy for me to eat.

A chicken is a bird. It has a head, body, wings, and legs and a tail. It has all white feathers all over its body. It walks on the ground and can't fly like other birds. People cut off its body parts of their head and feet, to eat the bird called wings, chest, thigh, and legs. Can you look at the computer or phone on the internet search for picture of a chicken to see what they look like?

Vegan Friends

I met someone, and he told me that he was a Vegan, and he said that he didn't eat animal meat, or drink dairy milk drinks and eat milk foods of cows.

He told me, that he sold his expensive car, because it had leather seats in it. He sold his leather car, because he found out that leather is animal, and he didn't want to own a car that was had animal leather car seats and didn't want to sit on cows.

He also said that he didn't wear animal leather shoes.

He said that his family used to own a business of animals, and he had to capture the animals. He told me that he had a dream, that the animals went to him in his dreams, and cried asking him why he captured them, so he stopped doing that.

Because of him, I went home and looked through my items, and found some leather shoes and leather coat, so I threw them away.

I met another friend and she said that she was a Vegan, and that she didn't eat any animal meat, or dairy milk foods.

She made me some carrot juice, and gave it to me to drink. I liked it. She also blended, some figs, and flax seeds, and gave it to me to drink. I drank them, and I liked it. She taught me about juicing and blending foods to drink. I used to juice for years, now I don't juice, I drink water and eat the foods from plants and trees.

My friend, had me meet her friend, and he who told me that he was a vegan also. He told me that he didn't eat fish, and that he didn't eat cow meat,

He said that he weighed 399 lbs. and that he died on the operating table. He asked a question when he died, "Why am I dying at age 39?"

He said he then saw about 50 people eating at a table. He looked, and asked the question in his mind, "Where is the milk and honey?" The people there replied back to his, "We do not partake of those things here." Then the vision opened up more, and then he saw the people, with the animals around them. When he came back to life he said, "Get me the dietitian. "Nothing must die, that I may live."

He showed me his large clothes, that he used to wear, yet now he lost all of that weight, and is average weight now.

He told me that he sold his dairy farm ranch and went Vegan. Now he teaches people how to be Vegan. He also teaches at farm stores, and at fairs, about being a vegan.

He gave me a juicer, and so I started juicing. I juiced for years and now I don't juice. I drink water and eat the foods from plants and trees.

That was three Vegans that I met. So, from those people who were vegans, I got informed about that Vegans didn't eat meat or dairy milk, nor did they wear animal leather, or use animal foods.

I didn't even know, that kind of vegan eating people existed, of not eating animal meat and dairy milk foods. I was not eating some meat and milk. And now I know that not eating all animal's meats, and not eating all dairy milk foods, is called being a vegan.

I was in my kitchen thinking about my life, and how I met three vegans. So, I asked a question out loud, "Should I be a Vegan?" I went Vegan in 1998. I made the decision to not eat all animal's meat, and not eat all dairy milk items.

Because of these people, being vegans, I learned from them. I wanted to be vegan like them, and now I'm a vegan.

Dairy Milk Items: milk, butter, cheese, cottage cheese, sour cream, ice cream, and chocolate

After meeting three vegans, I went to my refrigerator, and looked in, and saw dairy milk foods of animals. I decided to throw away of all the dairy milk foods of animals that I had in the refrigerator. I quit eating and threw away the butter, cheese, cottage cheese, sour cream, and chocolate that I had in my apartment.

I used to eat butter a lot, and it was difficult for me when I quit eating butter, because I thought about it for about the first week. I used to eat it, and now I wasn't eating it at all. I missed butter, yet I didn't eat it any more for health reasons. That was animal food.

Instead of butter, I started to use olive oil and that was a nice replacement, for me to use on my food. Then I found butter at the food store that was made from olives, that is dairy free with no animal milk in that, plant based.

It was different, to not have meat or dairy products, in my refrigerator any more.

Dairy is a name for cow's milk from it's utters, a female body part, where they pump the milk for drinks and for food with a silver milking machine. Could you not drink milk, or eat milk foods from cows or goats? And drink water, and eat water foods of fruits and vegetables.

Fish Meat

One day I was in my kitchen, and I thought about fish. I knew that fish, was the next animal, to stop eating. I hadn't eaten fish, in many years, since I was a child. For some reason, I thought about fish, that day and I made the decision, to not ever eat fish. And I didn't eat fish after that decision.

Sometimes I've seen fish, in the store behind the glass on ice, and I thought that is wrong and sad, because fish belongs in the ocean, in the water, not food for we to eat. I thought the fish looked sad there, where it's not suppose to be. I knew for me, that I would not be eating fish. I don't know if I ever ate fish, I don't think I did and if I did, it was only one time when I was a child. So stopping eating fish.

A fish lives in the ocean in the water. It has a head, body with scales on it, fins, and a tail. It swims in the water all day and all night. People catch the fish and cut off its body parts of its head, fins and tail, to eat the center body, called halibit, or salmon, of fish, fish sticks.

Could you look at the computer or phone internet search, and type in or say, picture of a fish, and see what a fish looks like? Could you not eat fish?

Shrimp Meat

I thought I ate shrimp at a party because I saw it there, yet I don't think I ate it. I stopped eating shrimp. It has been many years, since I ate shrimp. I thought I ate it with the red sauce. I didn't know, that they took off the head and the many legs off the shrimp, and left the tail on, and I ate the shrimp, that is wrong and sad I think. So, I shouldn't be eating shrimp.

Shrimp have a head, many arms and legs, body, tail. Pink in color. They live in the ocean waters and on the land. People take apart the shrimp and eat the body, not the head, arms and legs or tail. Could you not eat shrimp?

Could you look up on the computer or phone internet search and type of say, picture of a shrimp, to see what it looks like?

Crab Meat

I thought that I ate crab once at a restaurant, because it was expensive. After that I didn't eat it. I realized it was wrong and sad, to eat crab and I thought that I wish I never ate it. I think I just thought I ate it, yet I didn't eat crab. Crabs have a shell with many legs.

Crabs have a head and body, claws for arms, and many legs. They are grey in color. They live in the ocean and on land. People break open the body of the crab and eat it, and break open the legs, and eat the legs of the crab. Could you not eat crab?

Could you look at the computer internet search and type of say picture of a crab, to see what it looks like?

Lobster Meat

I never ate that. I saw them on the menu. I saw them at the restaurants life, and I sensed sad because I knew they cooked the lobsters in hot water, and they die from that, yet I never ate one.

Lobster has a head, body, claws for arms, many legs, and a tail. It's red in color. It lives in the ocean water and on the land. People take apart the lobster and eat the tail. Could you not eat lobster?

Could you look at the computer internet search and type or say, picture of a lobster, to see what it looks like?

Bee Honey liquid

I was in my kitchen, and I thought about bee's. I thought "What if a bee was given a bowl, and the bee spit in the bowl, and mixed it with the pollen, and called it honey, would I eat it?" No. I thought that the bee spits out saliva mixed with pollen, for its larva baby to eat, not for people to eat. Taking honey is stealing from the bees labors of their food for their babies. So since about 2001, I stopped eating honey.

Years later I was drinking an alovera drink, and about half way through, I decided to read the ingredients. To my sadness, the drink said that it contained honey. I immediately stopped drinking the drink, and threw it away. I thought oh no all those years of not eating honey, and I accidentally drank honey, in the drink that I bought.

I realized how important it is, to read the ingredients, so that won't happen again. The drink was an alovera drink, and it looked like water. They didn't advertise that honey was in the drink, on the front of the bottle, yet the small print on the back of the bottle, that said it contained honey. I didn't buy that drink ever.

Bees have a head, body, arms, legs, and wings. They are black and yellow. They fly to flowers to collect pollen, they put the pollen on their legs, and bring it back to the hive, mix the pollen with saliva for their babies to eat. Could we not eat honey from bees?

Could you look at the computer internet search and type or say, picture of a bee, to see what it looks like?

Juicer Machine

I went visit a vegan friend, and he gave me a juicer that he bought, so I gave him the money for it. That was my first juicer, and I began juicing right away almost every day. I juiced carrots and drank them. And I juiced cantaloupe and drank that. I juiced for years. And then my family said I was loosing the nutrients in the food by juicing. And I thought about it. I thought that the food doesn't spin in circles in a garden or farm on the land, they are sill for months on the trees or on the plants. So, I threw away my juicer and blender. I stopped that. And now I drink water mostly. From bottles or containers and pour the water into a glass, so I don't have to drink words on the bottle, to have new water.

Food Book

A friend of mine, told about a book she read, about food and the Essenes. The next day, I went to the book store, and found the book, and I started reading it. The book had so much truth in it. I read about how the Essenes were a certain people who ate from the table of the earth and land. They didn't eat animals, they didn't cook their foods, and they lived far away, from large cities, and lived on the land.

As I was reading that book, in the kitchen, I said to myself, "Where has this book been all of my life?" I had just found the book, and I had wished that I had read it a long time ago. I knew the book talked about the truth, about eating the garden and farm foods, new of the earth and land. It was a powerful book, and from reading it, I decided to do what the book taught, to eat my foods all new, not cooked. I thought that what the book taught, is what I want to be like, eating only new foods.

I got all of the cooked foods, that I had in the kitchen, in the cupboards, and threw them away. I wanted to try, eating only new foods, of the earth and land.

I thought that eating only new foods. I thought that being a new food person is even higher than a vegan, because vegans eat cooked foods, and the essenes in the book, only ate new foods uncooked. I thought I would try this way of eating new foods, being a new food person. It was 1999, when I made that decision to eat all new foods.

I ate and juiced a cantaloupe for breakfast, a banana for a snack, salad for lunch, nuts for a snack, and carrot juice for dinner. I felt nice, free, and fine.

Vinegar Fermentation

I was eating an oil and vinegar salad dressing on my salad, because most of the other salad dressings, have milk in them.

What will it do to me, if I don't eat vinegar? So, I stopped eating vinegar. I only used olive oil, on my salads, and sometimes some lemon. I liked it, and it seemed to be better on my salad, and more natural without the vinegar. The salad seemed to taste more new.

I decided to stop eating vinegar fermentation, in 2012. After a while of only using olive oil, I tried the Italian dressing again, and after I ate that salad, I noticed that stomach felt sick. So I knew that the vinegar wasn't for me to eat, and I went back to using the olive oil on my salads.

And then, sometimes I only eat the salad plain, without any olive oil, to try spinach and lettuce, the way it is in its natural form, of the garden and farm new.

Citric Acid

I used to eat a lot of green olives, and one day I read the ingredients, on the label of the olives, and it said citric acid. I didn't know what citric acid was, and I didn't think that it was needed. So I read on the internet that citric acid is a preservative and it ferments the foods.

I stopped eating olives, pickles, and yellow peppers, because they all have citric acid, in the water, and then the citric acid then gets into the foods. I thought, I would try not eating olives, pickles, and yellow peppers, any more just to see what it would do. I missed the olives because I ate a lot of olives, yet I did notice a taste to them that made them not new, and sometimes I felt sick from eating them, so I stopped eating them.

I don't want to eat citric acid, since it is used to sour foods. That preservative changes the natural new form, of the foods from a new way, to a fermented way, that is old, and that is not new garden foods.

And if the foods have to be preserved with citric acid, then the food is old, and not new. The natural enzymes in the foods are depleted, and the food no longer has its natural value, of new.

I stopped eating the citric acid olives in the jars, and I did find black olives in a can filled with water and ate those.

Vegan Clothes and items: Coat, Shoes, Wallet, Belt, Pillow, Blanket, Sofa, and Chair

One day my vegan friend told me he didn't wear leather shoes. So, After, I became a vegan, I went through my clothes, and realized, that I had to throw away my black leather coat, that I had bought and worn. I don't know why I bought a leather coat, because it was the social thing to do, I thought, at the time. I saw stores that had the leather coats, and I didn't know about not wearing animal leather from cows, at the time. So I threw away my leather coat, because I realized that it was animal leather, and leather is cow item. Now I wear fabric coats of fleece, linen, and cotton.

I also, threw away my leather shoes, and started looking for man made materials shoes, and vinyl shoes at the shoe stores. I found some and bought a few pairs that I liked. Once I bought some shoes, that I liked and wore them, yet they seemed to make me walk wrong. I wondered if they were leather, so I went back to the store, and read the box, and realized that they were genuine leather. I had forgotten to read the box, and I thought that they might be vinyl, yet they were not. I threw the shoes away, and kept wearing my other vinyl shoes.

I had a black leather wallet, that I had bought, and I knew that I had to throw it away, since it was animal item. I had to keep my ID and money in my pocket, because there were only leather wallets. Now, years later, I found a fabric wallet, and bought it at the mall. I was there at the right time, and I really like the fabric wallet. That store is not there anymore so I found it in time. Years later I found a vinyl wallet at the store and purchased that.

I had a leather belt and threw it away, and bought a vinyl belt.

I had a fabric sofa, and later I had a leather sofa. That was before I was a vegan. And I didn't know about leather and what it was. I didn't know that leather was animal skins of a cow, converted into covers for furniture of sofas, chairs. I didn't like that. My vegan friend said he would sit on a leather sofa. So, I couldn't sit on the sofa any more, it made me sad knowing that it was leather from cows bodies, so I threw it away, and got a fabric sofa again.

Throwing away those leather items of mine, was the right thing to do, once I knew about it. I shouldn't have had them, yet I didn't know not to, at the time. Now I do. And, I avoid purchasing anything, that is animal cow skins called leather that they take off of the animal's body. I don't want that in my house. I don't want to sit on cows. I want fabric furniture of sofas and chairs.

I had seen a chair at the store and I like it, and when I arrived at home I notice the chair had swans faces, carved into the wood with feathers, and spotted printed fabric like and animal. I had to throw it away.

I also had some imitation fur coats, many, that I wore often. Then I realized that the imitation fur looked too much like animals, so I threw them away. I bought cotton and fleece coats and vests from stores on the computer internet page.

After I threw away my leather items, I wasn't sleeping very nice so, I realized that I had other animal items, that I had to throw away. I started to notice that feathers were taken out of the blanket and I thought, "Birds." I didn't know what kind of bird it was from, and I didn't want birds in my bedroom on my bed. I had a bird feather down pillow, and bird feather down comforter bed cover. I really I liked them, yet I knew that I had to throw them away, since I was a vegan. So, I bought a fabric pillow and blanket and slept much better.

When I had the leather and feather items, I didn't realize that they were from animals. I just thought it was a coat, shoes, belt, wallet, pillow or blanket. I didn't think that they were all from an animals. When I went vegan, I got more conscious about food and items made from animals. I didn't want to ware or use a cow or a bird on my body or in my home on my items.

Vegetarian Friends

I did meet a vegetarian, and she ate a lot of salads like me. I told her that I was vegan, and that I didn't eat all animal's meat or dairy milk. I explained to her the higher way of living, of not eating all animal's meats and no dairy milk either, to inform her. I thought that if I told her what I did as a vegan, she could learn from me, and do the same maybe by becoming a vegan some day.

I met another lady who said she is a vegetarian and didn't eat some meat. I did the same thing, and told her I was a vegan, and explained that life way to her.

I was happy to meet vegetarians even thought they weren't vegan, maybe some day they will be vegan or new food people.

Gardens and Farms

In grammar school, we had to plant a sunflower seed, in dirt, in a paper cup. I poured water over it, and we put our cup in the window ledge, for the sun to lighten that seed. I remember looking down into the cup at the dirt, not seeing the seed. After a few days, I saw the seed popped up, from the dirt, like a sprout. I was happy, and this was my first experience, of growing something from a seed.

One day our family bought some dirt, and we made a garden in the back yard, a rectangular shape. My family showed me how to plant a garden. We dug a hole in the ground, put the plant in the hole, put the dirt back in the hole, and watered the plant. It was a tomato plant. I did that and I thought that was fun to do.

I helped plant the garden, weed, and pick the vegetables. We also planted fruit trees, in the back yard all around. So, I picked fruits from the trees in our backyard, and ate them. It was fun. We always ate salad every day, at dinner, and had fruit salads often.

I appreciate the garden and farm, of the foods that we planted there, and the garden has been an example in my life.

So when I moved away, and had my own, I planted a garden with tomatoes red and yellow, zucchini, peppers, corn, and beans. I planted rows of vegetables. I watered the garden a few times a week. The vegetables and fruit grew, and I ate the food right outside, in my garden, and that was nice. It was fun. I did some juicing fresh from my garden too. It was nice to be outside in nature as a farmer at my home in my back yard. I liked that.

The Food Store

When I to drive to the food store, I first shop to get my fruits and vegetables, all in the food store. Then I look for vegetarian and vegan foods in the cans. I get soups that are only vegetables. I got cookies, without any eggs, or milk, in them. I had to read every ingredient, to make sure, it was not animal items. And I had to find potatoe chips without any milk or cheese on them. I did this, as a vegetarian and vegan.

I have seen the meat and dairy milk areas, yet I don't shop there. I don't buy any animal's meat of: cow, pig, fish, lamb, shrimp, crab, lobster, bee honey, or egg.

I don't buy any dairy: butter, milk, cheese, sour cream, cottage cheese, yogurt, chocolate, whey or ranch.

And I don't buy honey, vinegar products, or citric acid products.

I try not to buy canned or boxed foods as they are not new foods.

As a vegetarian or vegan the canned vegetables and soups are ok, yet read all of the ingredients, to make sure that there is no, animal's meat or dairy milk, in them.

I can't eat cookies with animal items in them. I did find a vegan chocolate chip cookies, at the health food store, and I tried them.

I can't eat cake, because of the eggs, butter, and milk, in them, nor muffins, or croissants.

I ate fruit pie a few times, yet later I found out in the ingredients, they have eggs in the. I thought no eggs were in the fruit, it must be in the crust, so I cannot eat pie.

When I am shopping, I look at the food that I selected in the cart, and I see all of the fruits, vegetables, and nuts, that I selected, and it makes me happy.

When I am waiting, at the checkout stand, sometimes I see people, who have food on the counter, checking out, that is mostly all dead animal items like meat, eggs, and milk. I don't like seeing that, so I focus on what I have of fruits and vegetables, no animal meat or animal milk. I think it is sad that people eat that way, yet they don't know any better yet. Those foods seem to be dull, without any life in them, and no color. It's mostly a false family tradition of eating animals, that should be stopped. And start eating only garden and farm foods as a new family tradition.

I see that I don't shop the dead way. I shop the new food way. I don't buy animal meat or dairy milk items. And I am happy, for the new garden and farm foods, in my grocery cart, that I can buy, to eat.

As I have practiced being a vegetarian, vegan, and new food person, if I ate something, and I found out later, that it had animal products in it, I don't eat that any more, and keep going with my garden and farm food commitment. I realize that I must read all of the ingredients, to make sure that there are no animal items in them. It's nice to eat the new fruit and vegetables, of the land and earth.

Fruits and Vegetables

Now, as a new food person, I usually shop, only in the fruits and vegetable area, where the new food is. I stand there and look out around, and see all the colorful fruit and vegetables, and it makes me happy. I have bought almost every kind of fruit, vegetable, and nuts that I have seen.

There are fruits that you can eat, or peal and eat, or cut and eat. I have tried the fruits that are pre cut for you, by the store, yet sometimes they are old and fermented. And someone else cut them, so I don't buy already cut up fruits any more. I like to prepare my own foods myself. I like to buy the new fruits and vegetables solid and cut them myself at home.

I stopped cooking potatos in the oven and I started to lightly steam the potato in the in a pot with water, to have it not so cooked. Yet now I eat sweet potatoes, and potatos, new, instead of cooking them. I like to eat them new, the sweet potato, it's like a carrot, yet sweeter.

When I ate animal foods of meat and milk foods and cooked foods I weighed more. And since I have eaten mostly new foods: fruit and vegetables, I have lost weight about 29 pounds.

I always seem to have energy and feel nice eating from the garden and farm foods.

New Food People, of Fruits and Vegetables

As a new food person, I have really liked eating daily, of only fruits and vegetables. I like to eat one fruit or vegetable, at a time, to get the essence of the food. I like to sense the energy from the food I eat. I eat fruits and vegetables, every day, to get a balance of the gardens and farms.

I don't juice a much as I used to, I eat the foods in their natural form, and drink water.

I stopped cooking my food for many years, and I ate fruits and vegetables solid or cut up.

I have been learning about food for 40 years, eating mostly garden and farm foods, and eliminating animal meat and dairy milk items. And I feel better. I plan to continue to eat mostly new food, for the rest of my life, eating only fresh fruits and vegetables, and water. And I'm a woman that eats new foods and who wants to be with a man who is only a new food person.

And to this day, 40 years later, from 1980 to 2020, I am still a Vegetarian, Vegan, new food person, not eating animals, and only eating foods from the gardens and farms.

Computer Internet

I have found some vegetarian, vegan, and new food, computer pages and team meetings, on the computer, to see that there are others out there, who believe in being a garden, and farm eaters. I have watched videos on how to make fresh food dishes. And I have watched about the business of animal's buildings, and what they do there, to cows, chickens, sheep, pigs, and goats. The videos show them milking cows and goats. And I watched videos showing the cutting up the cows, chickens, pigs, and sheep, for food. It's wrong and sad.

I'm happy to not eat animals. New foods are for me. That is the best way to be.

Food Thoughts

Since I have eaten as a vegetarian, vegan, and new food person, since I was 14 years old, I feel happy. I am now 54 and being a raw food person feels the best for me. It has been a learning process of eating better, and informing me, about the best way to eat foods.

I am happy, to have met people, who told me about the foods, that were made from animals body's, and animals milks was wrong and sad. I am happy, to have read books that talked about what foods to not eat, that are animal based.

I am happy, to have met vegetarians, and vegans, who were practicing and living, eating garden and farm foods, instead of animal items, and not wearing animal items either. They taught me how to continue, to do what I was already doing, not eating animals. I learned from people, and books about foods, and which ones were nice for me to eat.

I have been not eating animal items, since 1980. I have not been eating animals, and not wearing animal products, for about 40 years. Not eating animals, not wearing animals makes me feel better over the years. I feel better eating new foods, over cooked.

My stomach feels lighter and free. My body feels better, and I don't get sick, only if I eat cooked foods, I might feel heavy and tired. If I've made a mistake, and eaten something that I shouldn't have, that might milk or eggs in it, that I didn't know, I don't do that again. And I read all of the ingredients, if I eat vegan from something cooked that's ok, and I like to eat new foods the most.

And that is what I am doing, by writing a food journal, to explain to people, how I started, as a vegetarian, and became a vegan, and then a new food person. It's a process, and it took me years, to learn how to eliminate eating animals, and wearing animals, in a world that mostly eats animal's bodies meats, drinks animal's fluids milk, and wears the animal's skins leather clothes and shoes. In my world, I don't eat them or wear them.

So, I have met 3 vegans and 2 vegetarians in my life, and it is interesting, this life style, of not eating animals, or not wearing them. There are only a few of us, yet more are learning.

Seeds of Plants and Trees

It's important to not eat the seeds in fruits or vegetables. Cut out the seeds out of the tomatos and bananas. And it's important to not eat beans, since they are seeds, they grow seeds, not foods of plants. If we eat seeds, beans, they will sprout in you and grow spiritually. So leave them away from you. An apple once you take the seeds out, and eat the apple, it does not grow. The food of apples don't grow. The food to beans, and seeds all grow plants, and we shouldn't eat seeds, we should eat fruits and vegetables from plants and trees, of the land and earth and of our planet.

I cut out the seeds to a tomato and eat the tomato with out seeds. I cut the banana in half and knife out the small black seeds, and eat the banana without seeds. Could you cut and spoon out seeds in your fruits and vegetables?

How to be a
New Food People
Eating Fruit, Vegetables,
and Water

For Animal milk and meat, Vegetarians, Vegans, Juicing,
Blending, Food Processor, and New Food People

How to be from eating animals, and cooked foods,
to eating all fresh foods, of the garden and farms, of
the plants and trees, of the land and earth.

Health, Happiness, and Freedom

Information about Foods

Sharon Jacobs

First Day of the Year, and All Days

On the first day of the year, I wish that we could have a holiday in our cities and countries, of the world on earth of our planet, where everyone would only eat food, from the gardens and farms, of new fruits and vegetables, and drink water, on this day, all days, and every night, all around the world. Everyone, and animals, could only eat garden and farm foods, to see the earth and land, the gardens and farms foods, that nature and the earth made for us to eat. Imagine and realize this is excellent for us. We could all be new food people.

New food, fruit, vegetables and water are amazing. Food and water, is our energy, and supplies us with all that we need to live, and survive. What is your favorite food and beverage? It could be fruits and vegetables, with water. This is what is nice for we. When you drive or walk, to the food store, what do you buy? Do you buy from the farmers, who plant, water and harvest the food, for us to purchase and eat? Or do you purchase dead animal meat, and milk items that were not supposto eat and drink?

This food book is about learning of food, and what it does for us. This is the day to start being, a new food person, and have a nice life, in doing that, to change our life, and start a new way of being, eating healthy, and drinking healthy of only fruits and vegetables.

I wish we had a world, where we only eat garden and farm foods. Only eat fruit and vegetables, and water, and not eat any animal foods of meat or dairy milk. Give nature to us. Give the animals a rest, and respect them, and respect yourself, by not eating them. It takes courage and strength to stop eating animals, and eat fruits and vegetables only, for our mind, body, and spirit. Walk into the garden and farms, and walk that path of new foods, for a new day for you, and for we.

We mostly almost all are from a broken world of people, who ate animals, so let's make a new world, that is all with fruits and vegetables. We have the past, today, and the future tomorrow. The past was eating animals, so we can leave that world, and be in the now today, and eat fruit and vegetables only, and do this for our future forever.

If we could have the first day of the year, be a world where we only ate garden and farm foods, the world and earth would be a nicer place. We would feel better and live better. Then we could have all, the rest of the days of the year, be eating and drinking, garden and farm foods, in our lives. If we do this, we have achieved everything most important in our lives, because we eat every day, all through the day.

Trees and Plants Foods

Trees are powerful and strong. They grow tall. The trees produce new fruits. To eat from a tree gives us strength. Fruit helps us to grow and life. Plants grow from under the ground up, and they grow mostly vegetables and some fruits. We need a balance of trees and plants foods to eat. They absorb the day sunlight heat, rain waters, ground soil, air wind, and night coolness. So, if we eat fruits, and vegetables, from trees and plants, we too will be eating from the sunlight, water, air, and soil, and moon light that are in the foods, in the new foods of the land and earth.

Animal meat and milk foods don't grow. They are not strong. They are weak. Meat and milk are not from trees and plants. It is easy to pick fruit from trees, and pick vegetables from plants to eat. We can't pick fruit and vegetables, from a cow, pig, chicken, fish, crab, lobster, oyster, deer, or other animals. We are to not pick meat and milk from animals. We are to pick fruit and vegetables from trees and plants. We should only eat from trees and plants. We should not eat from animal's bodies called meat and milk.

Trees and plants are free, so eating from them, helps us to be kind. If you can, at home, plant fruit trees and nut trees, in your back yard and eat the fruit and nuts. Plant a garden or farm and eat the fruit and vegetables. You will like it.

We should build our body, from the fruits of trees, and vegetables of plants and trees. That will make our body strong and solid also. We should not make and build, our body, of weak dead animal's bodies meats parts and pieces, and animal's fluids milk drinks and foods. Meat and milk foods are from animals. We should also not build our body from cooked foods. Trees and plants are from the land and earth, and have been around for thousands of years. They have a history of making food for us of fruits and vegetables, and water. So build a body for the fruits and vegetables, to live in you, from the trees and plants.

We shouldn't use trees to build homes, trees are dead once you cut them down and cut the roots off of them, and cut the branches off of them they begin to die. So building a house of trees is building a dead house to live in, and termites eat the wood, so don't do that. If you have the money build your home from metal, and build your furniture from metal too. It is strong and lives, metal doesn't die. We shouldn't walk on trees wood floors, we shouldn't sit on trees wood chairs, and we shouldn't use trees for wood tables, or use wood for dressers. We should use metal frames for homes and furniture. And use plastic dressers. Save the trees to be for our food only.

Trees shed their leaves every year, they are without leaves for a while and grow new leaves. So our body can shed the animals we ate and shed the animals we drank, and get new bodies of flesh, bones, and organs, by eating only fruits, vegetables, and water.

If you eat trees fruits, you will stand like a tree.

Fruits and Vegetables, without the Seeds

Today is a nice day to start with healthy foods, from the garden and farms new.

Nature made the apples, cantaloupe, oranges, and grapefruits, that are round like the sun, moon, and earth. Carrots, celery, and zucchini, are tall like trees trunks or branches. Potatoes are like the mountains. So we should eat fruits and vegetables because they are like nature. Animal's meat is not like nature. Meat is man made from death of many animals. Fruits and vegetables are nature made of the land and earth, from soil, rain, sunlight, moonlight, and air.

Fruits of apples, plums, peaches, pears, raspberries, blueberries, and blackberries, you can eat directly. The skins are thin enough to eat.

Fruits you can peel like grapefruit, oranges, and banana, then eat. The skins are thicker and you cannot eat them, you have to peel them, and eat the fruit.

Fruits of cantaloupe, watermelon, green melon, that you have to cut with a knife to eat. And with the fruit you can eat, all of the fruit new without cooking them.

For vegetables there are foods that you can eat like tomatoes, sweet potatoes, potatoe, lettuce, cauliflower, broccoli, carrots, red or green peppers, green onions, that you can eat directly new.

Another vegetable you have to cut is avocado.

Nuts you have to break the shell off to eat the nut.

Fruits and vegetables supply us, with all that we need for health and energy to life. We don't need to eat animals to survive. We need garden and farm foods new for our mind, body, and spirit, and to our life on earth.

Fruits and vegetables have seeds in them. We should take the seeds out. Either way we have seeds to plant and grow new foods. Animals don't have seeds for us to plant and grow. Steak and chocolate candy bars, don't have seeds in them to plant and grow. That's why it is best to only eat foods that have seeds for us to plant and pick. This is best for our man and woman life.

Fruits and vegetables, all have roots from the plants and trees. They grow in the ground to be strong in nature on the land and earth. They all have leaves, and they grow up in the air, in the sunlight, rain, air, and moonlight. Animals don't have roots, the meat doesn't get sunlight, and rain, or soil. So meat and milk foods are not from nature, they are from animals. We need to eat foods with roots, leaves, and stems.

Fruits, vegetables, and nuts, have skins or shells around them. The skins protect the new foods. Some skins of fruits and vegetables, we can eat, and some skins of fruits and vegetables, we have to take the skins off and don't eat, it's a process to do that. We can learn from doing that. The skins of fruits and vegetables, makes our skin. Yet, people have taken the skins of leather, fur, feathers, and wool, off of the animals, to wear or use them for items, and we are not supposto do that.

New garden and farm foods, from the plants and trees, have wisdom, knowledge, and intelligence in them. They also have information that we need to learn, grow, and life. So after we eat them, sit still for a while, like the new food sat still and quiet, while they were growing for months. We can sit still for a few minutes, and absorb the stillness and quietness, of them and learn. Fruits and vegetables grow in a group or team on the tree or plant. Many grow together. Yet we eat them individually.

Fruits, vegetables, and nuts all new, will help you and your mind, body and spirit, to lose the animals meat and animals milk items, from you. They will change your body from animals, to garden and farms foods, from plants and trees.

Nature's trees and plants of fruits and vegetables, and water are like a school or university, where you learn information from. They are teachers, and they will teach you what you need to know, and help you with your life. They will give you knowledge and wisdom from the earth, and your life will be nicer than eating, drinking, wearing, and using animal's bodies called meat, and animal's fluids called milk. Eat fruit and vegetables, and drink water, instead.

It's nice that a tree and plant, can make fruits and vegetables, and they are treasures, and presents for us to eat. They will save we.

Fresh food of fruits, vegetables, and nuts are from the trees and plants, in the family of nature with the mountains, ocean, grass, flowers, sun, air, stars, and soil. Trees and plants of the land and earth, work for we, as they grow. If we eat them, we will be made from nature too. They are food of presents, from the trees and plants, with power in them, for us to eat. Animal's meat bodies and milk fluids are not presents, they are stolen man made items from the animal's life.

We must comprehend and understand with our minds, that we are to eat only fruits and vegetables, all new for we, and not eat the bodies of animal's meats, nor drink the fluids of animal's milks.

Man and Woman + eating fruits, vegetables, nuts = life, solutions, alive, health
Man and Woman + drinking water = life, solutions, alive, health
Man and Woman + wearing and using natures fabrics of cotton, linen, fleece, and vinyl = life, solutions, alive, health

Man and Woman + eating animals bodies of meat = dead, problems, sad, sick
Man and Woman + drinking animals milk items = dead, problems, sad, sick
Man and Woman + wearing or using animals skins of leather, fur, feathers, wool = dead, problems, sad, sick

On the farms and gardens, apples, oranges, cantaloupe, and other fruits are picked from the stems, of branches from trees and plants. Watermelon, potatoes, peppers, avocados and other vegetables are picked from stems from plants.

Meat and milk from animal's, are taken from animal's bodies meat and animals fluids milk. Animals don't grow on trees or plants, so don't eat them. Eat fruits and vegetables, and drink water.

If you need direction and guidance, if you are board, if you don't know what to do: eat fruits and vegetables, and water. It's right.

The garden and farms produce and grow fruits and vegetables, for us to eat day and night. They are outside for months every day and every night. So we should learn to take walks outside, more during the day, and take walks sometimes at night, to see what it's like to be a fruit or to be a vegetable in the light of day, and dark of night outside in nature, on the land.

Could you type into the computer internet, Fruits and Vegetables A to Z, and look at all the fruits that we could eat? Then say or type in, picture of fruits and vegetables, and look at all the many colors of the fruits and vegetables.

Nature is the law of our earth. Farms and gardens are the law, of growing food for people. Plants and trees is the law of eating, and water is the law of drinking. We must keep natures laws, to be free. We must realize this and do that in our lives.

New Foods of Fruits, Vegetables, and Water, are Made for Us

Garden and farm food, of the land and of the trees, are made for all men and women to eat. In the start of time, in the old days, when there were only two people on the earth and land, they lived in the garden and planted a garden and farm, of plants and trees, that produced fruits and vegetables. They ate the food from the plants and trees, new. They were farmers. They didn't cook their food. They didn't have blenders, juicers, food processors, refrigerators, stoves, ovens, toasters, can openers, spiral slicers, or pots, they only had their hand to pick the fruit, vegetables, and nuts, and eat them new.

The soil, sun, rain, moon, and air, all made the garden and farm foods for us to eat. They grew for months still and quiet growing slowly, yet the same every time. Garden and farm food was made for us, to eat for breakfast, lunch, dinner, and snacks. We can eat as much farm foods as we want, and feel free about that. Feel happy about that. Feel healthy about that. Food from the plants and trees are quiet, they don't make noise. We should learn from them to be more quiet in our lives, not so filled with noise from the radio or television.

Carrots and celery are long like arms, and legs, our bones in our body. Peaches, plums, grapefruit are like flesh on our body. Blueberries are like our eyes. Oranges and grapefruit have outer covering like our skin. A tomato is like our heart. String beans are like our fingers and toes. All food is related to the body and necessary for us to survive. As we eat living food of the plants and trees, we are living and alive, and do what is nice.

New foods of fruits and vegetables, have all the information of the world, land, earth, plants and trees, in them. So if we eat them we will have that information in we too. Fresh foods are examples, teachers, and leaders, of nature, of all the farms and gardens and of the land, earth, planet, world, and all of creation. They build and clean our body, and give we life. They help to cleanse out too much cooked foods, and animal items of meat and milk. They will create a new body for we, and change our dead body of animals, that we have eaten, to new garden and farm foods body. This is a new way of eating. Let's be patient, and allow the fruits and vegetables do the work for us, to cleanse our body, and give us a new body, full of life and living plants and trees foods.

What foods do you have in your body? Is that new garden and farm foods of fruits and vegetables? Or, is that animal's bodies called meat and animals fluids called milk? We will win if we eat and use plants. We will be sad if we eat, drink, wear, and use the animals.

New foods of only the gardens and farms, help us to rest, be still, and be quiet to have a more peaceful life. So, let's eat only new foods for we. Let's do that now, today, tomorrow, and forever, while we live on earth, and on the land. We need this.

Eating the fruits and vegetables and water, will lead out, the dead animals bodies flesh red blood, called meat, and lead out the alive cow white blood fluids, called milk, from the body. You will feel free and better. Keep eating new foods, of fruits and vegetables, to cleanse the body, mind, and spirit.

Colors of the Gardens and Farms Foods

The earth of nature was made with many colors: a blue sky and blue ocean, so eat blueberries. Green grass, is like green beans or green spinach or green apple. Green plants, and green trees, are like green leafy spinach, and green lettuce. A yellow sun, so eat yellow squash, cantaloupe, peaches. Night sky is dark like black berries. Flowers have many colors too, so eat fruits and vegetables that have those colors. Mountains are brown, so eat potatoes.

I like to eat of the gardens and farms, that have the many colors of the earth's rainbow like: yellow squash, orange oranges, red apples, green lettuce, blue blueberries, and black blackberries. Garden and farm fresh foods of fruit and vegetables, have a variety of color on them for we to eat.

Animal's products and cooked foods, that people have eaten, are a dull color. Not much color in dead food or cooked foods.

Today, I eat healthy. I eat the fresh fruit and vegetables, of the garden and farms, plants and trees, for breakfast, lunch, dinner, and snacks. I eat only of the natural earth, new foods of fruits, vegetables, nuts, and wheat, and I feel best doing that. They are living foods. I eat the foods that will help me better myself, of my mind, body, and spirit, to do what I do in life.

New Food Person

I have been a vegetarian growing up, and then a vegan, and now I am mostly a new food person. I like to say vegan, because some people know that vegans, don't eat animal items, or drink animal foods. I don't cook that much, and I eat mostly new fruits and vegetables.

Being a new food person, I have felt better, and I have liked my food more. The taste is better, and my body feels better, and it is nicer eating new foods for me. I went to the point of not even cooking my foods any more, because I only ate the fruits and vegetables new. I stopped cooking my food, blending, juicing, food processing, and spiral slicing my foods, with kitchen food machines. I ate like as if I was in the garden on the farm, pure and natural, of the land and earth. I wanted to see what it would be like, to live like they did, in the start of time, where they didn't have machines to cook foods. I wanted to eat my food just the way it was, in wholeness, still, and quiet. I felt better that way, and I lost 29 pounds, from not eating cooked foods any more, only eating fruits and vegetables.

When I eat cooked foods, as a vegan, I sometime feel tired, from the food, or sick, and sleepy. And that causes a problem for me especially during the day. When I was a child I was sick sometimes. I was sick from eating animals, yet as an adult vegan new food person, I don't get sick any more.

I like to learn about the food, and how it makes me feel. I want to learn, about how I can be a better person, by eating new foods, from the garden and farms, at the food store, or from my own garden. I can teach myself, and others, to be a new food person, and what foods are better for we, and how to do that.

Eating only new food is new. And you get to keep your body, if it is all fruits and vegetables. Yet if your body is made up of animal's meat and milk products, you don't get to keep your body. You must give back the animal's bodies to them. And how will you do that?

Could you be a new food person? They don't buy animal items to eat, they don't eat animal meats of: cows, chickens, turkey, pigs, fish, bee honey, shrimp, crab, lobster, lamb, goat, or other animals. They don't drink animal milk. They don't eat animal milk foods of: cheese, butter, yogurt, ice cream, sour cream, whey powder, ranch dressing, chocolate, or cottage cheese. They don't eat animal eggs. They don't wear animal skins of leather cow clothes, they use cotton, linen, fleece or velvet, vinyl materials and fabrics. They don't wear leather cow shoes, they wear vinyl or fabric shoes. They don't sit on cow sofas, cow chairs, cow cars, or cow motorcycles, they use fabric or vinyl. They don't use animal feathers, fur, imitation fur, animal fabric prints, animal pictures on fabric, or wool clothes, or items of animal's bodies skins.

The fresh food people eat fresh fruit and vegetables, not cooked. And if they do eat vegan cooked foods, they don't have meat, or milk items in the foods. They read the labels, of cans and boxes, to make sure that no meat, milk, eggs, whey, or butter, are not in the food. And they don't eat so much cooked foods, they eat more new foods, and drink mostly water. This is better for me, and for we. I thought that this might help, if you want to know about that.

Could you not eat animal foods, and eat only new garden and farm foods, of fruits and vegetables for two days, then a week and then a month? You can start with only new garden and farm, fruit of grapefruit for breakfast, and salad vegetables for lunch, and drink water, and have another fruit or vegetable for dinner or eat nuts. That is all. See if this works for you, a new way of life, for all of our lives. That is awesome and the nice way to life, more free and health conscious.

I know this way of eating works, because I have been stopping eating animals, and stop drinking animals, all of my life, one by one, as I learned about them. Someone told me about this, so I wanted to tell you. We could make our body, from the food of plants and trees, from the fruit and vegetables, instead of making our body from the dead animal's meats and milks, because animals are not food. The garden and farms of plants and trees, grows our food for we. This is nice for we.

There is only one way for me to eat, and that is fruits and vegetables only new with water. There is only one path for me to walk on in my life, and live, and that is eating only from the gardens and farms food, and shopping only in the food area. And I'm a woman with a man who eats only from plants and trees foods like me.

Being a fresh food person you own your body. Eating animals you don't own your body, because you put animals into your body and the animals own you. You have to give the animals bodies back to them, by not eating, drinking, wearing, or using the animals. You might have awards, trophies, collage degree, money, business of work, car, truck, motorcycle, boat, material possessions, an apartment, or a house, yet the most important thing that you can own, is your mind, body, blood, and spirit, filled with fresh fruits, vegetables, nuts, and water, from the gardens and farms, plants and trees, of the land on our earth planet.

Being a new food person, eating only new fruits and vegetables, and drinking water is the most human of eating style. You are an individual. Eating animal's bodies called meat, or drinking animal's fluids called milk, you are not all people, you are part animal and part people, not all the way one person, like a new food person is all one.

Most of us have been born, with animals, already in our body, from our parents, who ate or drank and ate animal foods. Then we grew up eating and drinking, animal's meat and milk, because of false traditions, of doing that in our homes with our families, and in restaurants. Yet you can make a change, and stop eating, drinking, wearing, and using animals, now today, and for the rest of your life. Rebuild your body. Build, maintain, design, and manage your body and spirit, with new foods of the land and earth, from plants and trees only forever on this earth and land where we have life.

Please stop eating, drinking, wearing, and using animals for food and clothes, cars, wall mounted plaques, items and accessories. Don't purchase dead animal's bodies parts and pieces of meat, and milk drinks. Please eat only new fruits and vegetables, and water every day, all day, for the rest of your life. Purchase only food from the farms and gardens. It's exciting to eat fruits and vegetables, and water. And I feel nice to eat like that. You will too feel nice to eat like that also.

New food people are leaders and examples, of how to eat of the farms and gardens, of the land and earth from only plants and trees. We have many choices to buy and eat only, of the food stores, from the farms and gardens. We have a variety to choose from. Try them all. Do this. And take out the seeds, don't eat the seeds of fruits and vegetables.

As a new food person, I walk, talk, sit, sleep, think, have relationships, work, and do other activities with new fruits and vegetables, in my body and spirit daily. I don't have animal's bodies of meat, and animal's fluids of milk products, in my body to do those things. I feel sad when I think about my family ate animals, and the city of people who ate animals. I feel happy when I think of vegetarians, vegans, or new food people, who try to eat mostly fruit and vegetables, and try to not eat animals. I feel happy when I think about the farm and garden foods, that I'm about to eat like an avocado, tomato, spinach, potato, apple, grapefruit, cantaloupe, grapes and orange. New food is necessary for my body, and spirit of my life. New foods affect me in a positive way, because I feel healthy. Animals and too much cooked foods, affect me and make me sick, so I don't do that any more so much.

Being a new food person, I'm building a better body and spirit for me. This is one thing I can control in my life, by eating only new foods of fruits and vegetables, from the farms and gardens, and not from the animals meat and milk drinks and milk foods.

I am the only new food person in my family, and I'm probably the only new food person in my city. And I have a responsibility to teach others what I know, to help them too. I wish we had more people who ate only new foods, from the garden and farms, in our world of people of fruits and vegetables.

I want to be with him who eats only new foods of fruits, vegetables and water. As I eat only fruits, vegetables, and water. Him and her. Who I'm supposto be with. Both new food people in this life.

Here's what I eat in a week as a new food person: grapefruit, orange, apple, cantaloupe, grapes, tomato, avocado, spinach, potato, and almonds. Take the seeds out, and drink water. I take out the seeds in the grapefruit and orange. I cut out the core of the apple seeds, I cut and spoon out the tomato seeds and not eat them. I spoon out the seeds of the cantaloupe. I take out the seeds of the banana. I eat those foods new every week.

From this book, I would like to start having, all the people of the world, land, earth, and planet, eat only of plants and trees foods. It's a solution of health and life for the world. It's a higher way of living and eating, at home, in the city, and in the world.

Farmers

Farms have one of the nicest work businesses on the land, in our city, earth, and planet. They farm our food in large gardens or farms on the land. They plant, water, wait, and pick the food, take it to the store, and sell it to all the people to eat. Farmers supply and give to we new fruits and new vegetables for every season of spring, summer, fall, and winter of the year. Their food is the healthiest, that we can eat. The food is still and quiet, all summer, and sits on the ground, or hangs from plants, and hangs from the trees. They are growing and waiting for us to eat it. Farmers give us the nicest of foods of fruits and vegetables, and water. Farmers have some of the most professional work business on earth.

I have a lot of respect for farmers, who plant my new foods. I only shop mostly in the fruit and vegetable area. My basket is filled up, with mostly all new fruits and vegetables. My refrigerator had only garden and farm food in it. I didn't have any animal items in my refrigerator, or grocery cart, home, or body, only garden farm foods. My kitchen counter is a place for my new foods to be, like in the gardens and farms.

Farmers work much to plant and pick our food, all year round, so we can have healthy new food to eat. Farmers have to wait for months, to get the food, from the trees and plants to harvest, pick, and sell in the grocery food stores for us. And yet we can have our new garden and farm foods, the same day that we drive to the store to buy it. We don't have to wait for months, the fresh foods that are already in the stores every day.

I like to try all of the different kinds, of fruits and vegetables, all new, not cooked And the farm and garden food from nature, of the earth, is guilt free, from not having to capture an animal, cut it up and eat it, and then get sick. So, I say thank you, to the farmers of the world, for all of the food that they work for, and sell to we, thank you.

Farmers are one of the nicest examples and leaders of the earth, land, farm, garden, fields, plants, and trees of fruits, vegetables, and nuts with water. They do this for the people, and they should be awarded for their efforts in that. Farmers know the path, that we should buy and eat, in our lives. We should follow the farmers, right to the food stores, and only buy from them our foods, and plant a garden or farm for ourselves. If you want to learn from someone, learn from the farmers who plant, water, harvest, pick, and sell fresh fruits and vegetables, of the land, to the people.

Farmers control 20% of the world's earth, land, farms, garden, fields, and trees to feed the people. The other 80% of food is controlled by people who cook the foods, and by hunters of the land, ocean, and air, of animals, and businesses of animal's manufacturers for food, drinks, clothes, shoes, and items. We need the farmers to be 100% in control of the world of food for the people. And we need to be 100% in control, of our purchasing power of food, and in control of our eating and drinking, from farmers only, new foods and drinks, to live all of our lives. Only buy from farmers, who farm our new food, and farm plants for clothes, shoes, and items.

What Foods do You Purchase and Eat?

What type of foods do you purchase at the food store? What kind of foods are in your refrigerator? What kind of foods do you put on your plate? What food do you set on your table? What foods are on your kitchen counter? What kind of foods do you put into your body? What food do you feed your family? What food do you buy at restaurants? Do you buy foods that are new, natural, full of color, sunlight, rain, soil, air, and moon light, from the farm and garden? Do you buy cooked foods? Or, do you buy dead animal foods, and drinks, that are dead, and processed?

Do you buy produce from the gardens and farms, new or would it be over cooked in the oven, stove, frozen, microwaved or dead foods that were cut up of dead animals? Maybe a change needs to happen. Change from buying dead animals bodies, of meat and alive animals milk dairy drinks and food, to fruit and vegetables? That's something to think about.

Fruit and vegetables, have water in them, and they grow with water. Dead foods have blood in them, as they are animals, and we don't want animal's blood or flesh, in our body. We only want water foods, in our body, that has supplied our foods with water to grow, from new fruits and new vegetables on the land, of plants and trees.

Maybe this is the year, to stop buying animal foods, and start buying new foods of fruits and vegetables only. Try something new. Try it, you might like it. I like that. This is the year to end viruses and this is the year to be healthy.

How do you want to start your year? This may be the day and year, to start eating only fruits and vegetables, and to try to stop eating so much cooked food, dead animal meat, and animal dairy milk drinks and foods. Have you ever done that before? Only eat new foods from the earth, instead of from cooked foods, or animal's body meat and dairy milk fluid?

There are four kinds of eating ways of people.

1. There are animal eaters who, ate animal items, that are dead cooked meats, and alive dairy milk drinks and foods.
2. There are vegetarians who stop eating some meat.
3. There are vegans who stop eating all meats, and all dairy, yet they eat cooked foods.
4. There are new food people who eat mostly, or only new foods. They don't eat cooked foods so much, and they don't eat meat, or dairy milk drinks or dairy milk foods.

Eating animal's items, makes us sick, overweight, and slow. Not eating no animal meat, and no animal dairy milk, is the better for we. And, eating mostly all fruits and vegetables, is the nicest for we. This is what I do. I used to eat some animal meat and animal milk foods when I was a child, yet I learned from other people, from a few books, and from myself, to not eat animals, to not drink animals, and to not wear animal's leather skins, and to eat only garden and farm foods. So I learned and heard of this, and read of this way, of eating and living, and I accepted it right away, and took action, to choose to do this, and I did. I like it. And I want to teach others, how to do the same. They need to know. I must teach others, to not eat animals. Maybe they didn't know, they were eating animals, all of their lives, and it's time to do something different, like eat only garden and farm foods, from the plants, and trees. Inspire by example.

Purchase to eat grapefruits, oranges, apples, cantaloupe, tomatoes, potatoes, and water to drink, every week. Take the seeds out of them, could you not eat the seeds? This is health.

New Foods, of Fruits and Vegetables

Eating new food all day of fruits and vegetables, is the nicest path, to eat throughout the day and life. You will feel you're nicest. The garden and farm food is there for we, to eat every day, to make our lives, the nicest that they can be. We need the living foods, that affect us in a positive way, to help we with our living life, while we are on this earth, and planet in the universe.

The cooked foods, processed foods, canned foods, boxed foods, frozen foods, refrigerated foods, or animal foods is usually not the best for we, and can affect we in a negative way, where the living foods, will affect we in a positive way. Fruit and vegetables are living food. Cooked food and animal meat and milk items, are dead foods. We want to eat living foods, because we are a living people.

Most vegetarians and vegans, try to eat more fruit and vegetables, yet they still eat the cook foods sometimes. The new food person, eats more new and living foods only, not cooked foods, and not old foods that are fermented. They also think, that the new foods, of the garden, and farm is better for them. All vegetarians, vegans, and new food people, are more health conscious, and really watch what they eat, to make sure it is healthy, and more of the garden and farm foods, than meat or dairy milk drinks or foods. They read the ingredients. New food doesn't have ingredients. They are nice and true. They are awesome for we to eat.

Animal meat and animal milk items have blood in them. Fresh produce of fruits and vegetables have water in them. We need as much water, as we could, to feed our body daily. And new foods have minerals, vitamins, enzymes, protein, calcium, fiber, energy, and color.

Stop Eating	Start Eating
Cow meat	New Fruits
Pig meat	New Vegetables
Chicken meat, chicken eggs, Turkey meat	Purified Water
Fish, crab, lobster meat	
Any Other Animals	
Cow or goat milk	

How easy is it to eat garden and farm food? Simply walk to a tree, and pick the fruit, wash it, dry it off, and eat it. Healthy, and full of life. Freedom is in this. This is the path the universe was designed to be. Our food is to be from, the garden and farms, of the land and of the earth. Not from the animals bodies, or milk fluids drinks, and milk foods.

Fruit are solid. Vegetables are solid. Fruit and vegetables have a stem that you pick off. They don't have a head, arms, legs, tail, fur, feathers, wool, or blood. Fruit and vegetables, and nuts have water in them. And we need water to live. Animals walk on the land. Garden and farm food don't walk, they are still and quiet as they grow. Fruit and vegetables hang from plants and trees, they sit on the ground, or in the ground.

It's so easy to buy a fruit tree, plant it in your back yard, and pick the fruit when it's ready, wash it, dry it, and then eat it happy and free. It's so easy to buy vegetable plants, plant them in your garden, in your back yard. And pick the vegetable when it's ready, wash them, dry them, and eat them happily, guilt free, because it has no blood in them, only water.

With fruits and vegetables, you don't have to think what it is, or where it came from. It came from a tree, or from a plant, grown in the earth, with soil, rain and sunshine. No life was taken in the process, of picking fruits and vegetables. You only cut the stems to get the food, and take out the seeds to plant, in the land in nature. To get meat from an animal, they had to death them, cut their body all up to do that, and there are no seeds to plant to grow another animal, once the animal is gone, it's gone. No seeds from the animals to plant to grow another animal.

Sometimes looking at animal meat, you don't know what it is, all cut up in pieces. It's an animal. You always know what you are getting with fruit, vegetables, and nuts. Even when you cut them up, you still know its garden and farm food.

We are to plant and pick fruits and vegetables, to eat for our body. We are not to plant and pick animal's bodies, and fluids to eat for our body, or drink for our body. We are to touch fruits, vegetables, and nuts with our hands. We are not to touch the animals.

Look at all the variety and different kinds of fruits and vegetables, all fresh for we to eat daily. I make the healthy choice of eating that path, on my path in this world of life, as a new food person.

Farm and garden new foods are still as they grow for months. Eating fruits and vegetables, helps us to be more still in our lives. To sit in silence when you eat your food is nice. Sit in the quiet, of the farms and gardens, where the new food grew. It's a food relationship with the fruits and vegetables eating them. As you are in the quiet eating new foods, you can learn from them. They are teachers, of the land and earth. Eating fruits, vegetables, and water, all help us to have energy and life. We were made to eat on this path, for all of our lives, for breakfast, lunch, and dinner, every day and forever.

Eating

When we are eating food, it is nicest to eat in the quite peace, of the place where we are eating. No television or radio should be on, because we should like the peace, of the room, and like the food of itself, and with our family, or by ourselves.

We should focus on our food, that we are about to eat, into our body, and let the quiet be important, for us to sense. We should keep our talking to a minimum, or not at all. We should bond with our food, to let the food teach us, what it is about, and how it can help us with our lives.

We should be sensing the energy, sensing how we are supposed to feel, with our new food of fruits and vegetables, as we prepare them to eat, and clean up, and relax after we eat.

Breakfast is important for our day. Eating fruit is best for us. Fruit is all we need for breakfast. Eating one fruit, is enough to make it, for the next several hours. Eating one fruit like a grapefruit or a potato is plenty. It is easy to prepare and eat.

You may see how that fruit helps you, in the morning throughout the day. You will feel best eating only fruit. You could eat more fruit and vegetables.

Try to not eat cooked foods, and only eat the fruit. If you need to eat cooked foods, keep it to garden and farm foods, and not meat or milk drinks, or milk foods from cows. Try doing this for a week, to see how you feel in your body, mind, and spirit, at work, or at home.

Lunch is important to help us, through the rest of our day. So, eat only new vegetables, like a tomato or avocado. See how you feel for the day. Only eat vegetables plain how they are, and remember, that you ate fruit for breakfast, so now you need a balance of vegetables for lunch.

For Dinner you could eat fruit, vegetables, or nuts. Fruit may be more light feeling for you.

Have one day where you eat only new foods, as an experiment just to see how you feel, eating that way. It will be a nice day.

Eat One Food at a Time

Eating one food at a time, is the right way to eat. Like eating only a grapefruit, for breakfast, and that is all. Eat only an avocado for lunch and see how you sense. See what the food does for you, alone by itself. You can experience what the food does, the energy it has, and how the energy works for you. Eating one food at a time is more pure, and will be healthy for you. You will get to know the food better. I have a food high from eating the food new, not cooked. When I eat cooked foods, I don't get that food high. I feel more tired, and my stomach hurts, from eating cooked foods, and slow. That's why I like to eat my food new, to experience me with the food, that's new and to experience nature.

Sometimes I like to eat one food at a time, and see what that is like doing that. And then after I have ate only one food for breakfast, I like to eat only one food for lunch, to see what that is like eating it alone.

At times I will eat two foods together, either all fruit, or all vegetables. I try not to mix the foods together too much at meals. I like to eat either all fruit at a meal, or all vegetables at a meal. I try to keep my eating of food nice, and pure of new fruits and vegetables.

Awake

Eating as a vegetarian, vegan, and fresh food person, I realized that I am more awake, than others, in my eating habits. I can see that I eat healthier, and that I have more respect for the animals, by not eating them, meat, and by not drinking them, milk. I learn in eating on the path I should. When I hear about not eating an animal, I stop eating it. I learned that eating meat and dairy milk is wrong and sad. So, I stop and listen, and start to do what I need to do for myself. I can't save them from eating wrong and sad foods, if they don't want to, and I wish they did want to save them selves. I can only save myself, from eating wrong and sad foods, and try myself to eat the nicest that I can, of the right foods. When people told me animals were made into food, I didn't want to eat them anymore. Sometimes when I tell people, "I don't eat animals", they say they can't do that. I think to myself, "I don't want to eat animals." And I don't.

I wish I had a family that taught me from birth, to child, to adult not to eat animal's bodies meat, not to drink animal's fluids milk. I wish they told me to not cook my foods, and eat them new and alive instead of dead foods. I wish my family was more awake and ate vegetarian or vegan. They eat meat. I'm the only one in my family, that doesn't eat animal meat, and animal dairy milk drinks, and dairy milk foods. I think that they are older than me, and they are still sleeping, in their awareness of eating animals. I am awake, and I keep awakening, because I don't eat animals, nor drink animals. I eat and drink garden and farm foods. I like being awake to that realization.

I know what to do, about the way I eat, and what is nice. If I'm at a dinner, where people all bring food to eat, I have noticed that most of them, bring food that has meat, or dairy in it. So, I have to look for the salad, vegetables, and fruits. And I have to really look, at the salad, and vegetables, to make sure, that there is no meat in that.

It is something that I have noticed, of how most people, around me, have been eating and drinking, animal foods, and I eat earth food, in the world I live in. People have taught me how to eat that way by tradition, and I have to live in my own life, with my own way of eating and thinking, and start my own new traditions, and eat my own habits, even if I do that alone.

I think that there must be some vegetarians, or vegans, and new food people, out there somewhere. So I have found some videos, on the computer, and watched them talk, about eating and drinking healthy. And I have read magazines, that I ordered about eating new foods.

I live mostly on my own about eating like this, even around others, I know that I am different, and I like being different. I wish that there were more people, who ate vegetarian, vegan, and new food people, in the world. All I can do is be an example of this, and maybe the people around me, will notice, and make a new change, for them selves, and for the better.

I woke up to, when I found out, that animals were made into food. I was sleeping about not knowing, about that. So I became a vegetarian for years.

I woke up being a vegan, finding out that there were people who didn't eat, drink, or wear none of animal's meat, and milk items, and animal clothes. I was sleeping to that, I didn't know, now I know.

I woke up being a fresh food person, eating only from the garden and farms, of fruits and vegetables, new and uncooked. I didn't cook my food any more, I ate the fruits and vegetables alive, not dead foods. I was sleeping to that awareness. Now I'm aware and awake. I wish I could have been awake for all of my life, yet it took years to learn, about what foods to eat all new, and I learned about what animals to not eat. None of them. And now I know.

And I recently learned to not eat the seeds in the vegetables or not to eat some nuts or seeds, because they grow. If I eat an apple they don't grow when you eat them, only when you plant the seeds in the ground, and water them they grow. I wish I would have known to not eat the seeds of a tomato and banana, a long time ago, I would have never don't that. So I'm awake to that realization.

New Path

What kind of foods do you eat when you are alone, with your husband or wife, family, or around other people? Do you eat what they are eating, or do you eat what you know you should eat: vegetarian, vegan, and new food habit. Like a salad, and fruit, with water.

Most people have grown up, eating some fruit and vegetables, and mostly cooked foods, animal meat and animal milk drinks and animals milk foods.

As a vegetarian, vegan, and new food person, I have to change what I used to eat, to a new way of eating. I must be careful what I eat. Most of the world of people's path of eating habits, has been eating animal's bodies meat and drinking animal's fluids milk. I don't do what is the old way, of eating animals. I do the new way of eating, only from the garden and farms, of plants and trees. I may be the only one, yet I know this is right. I have mostly been alone in being a vegetarian, vegan, and new food person. Not many people know about that.

I have to ask questions, to the waitress, about what is on the menu, or in the food? I need to know about the ingredients to make sure, that there are no animal foods, in my food. Most menu's are sad with all of the animals meats and milks on them, yet, if they have one salad, and a few side orders of like potatoes, broccoli, and fruit, otherwise than that, the entire three page menu has been mostly animal items, of animals of all kinds, prepared in all different ways.

So find the salad, on the menu, with only vegetables on that. And find some fruit for dessert.

Be different from the old way of the world. Create your own world of fresh foods. Create a new path for you in your home.

Energy

After you eat your food, stay sitting, and rest, think, and sense how you feel, after you have eaten your food. You can really feel the energy of the food, working in your body. Take a walk is nice with that energy, or to do something around the house, or in the yard, or relax.

It's important to think about the food, that you have eaten, or about the food, that you will eat. Eating is very important several times a day. We should think about what foods, that are nicest for us, like new fruits, fresh vegetables. All the garden foods have energy stored inside of them. They are ready, to give that to we.

All new foods, of fruits and vegetables, are in the food store, they are nice for we, not cooked so much.

Lightly steamed is better, than cooked too much, microwaved, frozen, oven, or stoves. A pot with warm water lightly steamed, is to keep the minerals and vitamins, in the foods, and not cook the enzymes out. Don't cook out all of the nutrients and fiber, in the foods, even the color changes, cooked in the vegetables and fruit, if you cook them too much. Could you not do that? Could you not eat them cooked and cut them up, and eat them new?

We need the energy, from the new fruits and new vegetables. They have energy from the trees, energy from the rain, energy from the soil, energy from the moonlight, energy from the air wind, and energy from the sunlight. We run out of energy, if we cook our foods, or eat animal foods of meat and milk. Animal meat and milk foods have no energy. They have no sunlight, no moonlight, no rain water, no soil, and no air wind. There is no oxygen air, or water, in meat and milk drinks or milk foods, because there is mostly red blood in meat, and white blood fat in meat, and white blood fluids in milk, all of that in the animal meat and animals milk.

And we need energy and oxygen air, to live and function, and we get that from the new foods on plants and trees, from the land of the earth and planet. There is no energy and oxygen air or water in animal's bodies, called meat or in animal's fluids called milk. Thats dead foods. So eat alive foods of new fruits and vegetables.

Our Body

What kind of body do we have, and what kind of body will we have, at the end of our life? How are you building your body? With fresh garden foods, of fruit and vegetables? Or are you building your body, with dead, lifeless animal's parts and pieces of their bodies?

Imagine your body laying there in the grave, and you are a spirit in heaven, in the spirit world of people. We won't be eating animals in heaven. They only eat fruits and vegetables there. So why wait to die, and get to heaven, only to find out, that no one eats animals there. It's better to know now, that they don't eat animals in heaven. No meat or dairy is served there. So you'll miss it. So miss it now. Start now not eating meat or drinking dairy milk drinks from animals, because just like us when we die we will be a spirit without a body. The animals will be spirits, with no bodies for us to eat. So, we will have to eat fruits and vegetables only.

You have to become a new food person in heaven. So why wait? Why not be a vegetarian, vegan, or new food person now? And if you eat only garden and farm foods here on earth, and in heaven, what will you think of your body laying there, for years, all filled up with animals, broken body parts and pieces, like a dead zoo of animals?

Shouldn't we build our body, from the garden and farms, of trees and plants, instead of from animal's flesh meat bodies, and animal's milk fluids drinks? Yes. After I die and get my body back, I want to be back into my body, that has been eating only garden foods, from the farms of trees and plants. I don't want to be back into a body, that is all filled up with dead animal's bodies. That would be wrong and sad. So I have to start now, every day, to eat only, from the land and earth, to build my body, and protect my body from dead foods. I need to eat life foods full of sunlight, moonlight, soil, air wind, and rain water of fruits and vegetables new.

Are you building your body, with garden and farm foods, life from the earth and land made by nature? Or, are you building your body, with dead animals from the business of animals made by men? What materials are you using to build your body? Do you build your body and spirit with dead animal's meat and animal's milk drinks, or alive materials of fruits and vegetables?

When I ate animals, it changed my body system, I got sick and had a virus. I couldn't do it any more. I don't like feeling sick. When I started eating only new foods of fruits and vegetables only, I didn't get sick and I was healthy.

Do you have fruit and vegetables in your body? Or do you have dead animals in your body? I don't want dead animals in my body. I want garden and farm foods, from threes and plants, in my body, every day, for all of my life.

Do you have a relationship, with garden and farm foods, of plants and trees, fruits and vegetables, in your body? Or, do you have a relationship, with dead animals in your body?

Look at Food

As you are studying to be a vegetarian, vegan, or new food person, eat the new fruits and vegetables, and water as much as possible. Do this for breakfast, lunch, dinner, and snacks. Could you not cook your food as much, or not at all, and take walks? Shop only in the new food area for food. And find restaurants, that serve a lot of fruits and vegetable. Could you eat the food, at room temperature, since it was grown outside in the natural light, air, water, and soil of the earth and land, at nature's temperature?

Think about garden and farm foods, when you are hungry, and try to find fruit to eat, at connivance stores. Let people know, that you are a vegetarian, vegan, or new food person, and how you eat, so they will learn about it, and maybe they will do the same, as you. Let them know how you eat, so that if they are cooking or making food, they can make something for you to eat, that is new food.

Keep a fresh food journal, for yourself, for a while to write, what you have been eating, and what you want to eat now. Find some magazines, books, and computer pages, that teach about eating healthy new foods. And like being a vegetarian, vegan or new food person.

When you are at the food stores, look at the food. Look at all the variety of colors. Try to buy many different sorts of fruits and vegetables. I stopped using salt. Instead I eat the foods the way they are, to have the natural salts in them. I like to eat my fruits and vegetables.

Information

We eat three meals a day. We eat food every day for breakfast, lunch, and dinner. We have to eat, to feel nice and stay alive. Food is very important. And the kind of food we eat, should take much consideration. We should only eat fruits and vegetables and water every day.

We should never eat any animal's, meat or dairy milk drinks from cows or goats, at all during the day or night, because the blood in the meat and milk gets into our bodies, and we get sick with the Coronavirus from cows, goats, pigs, turkeys, chickens, fish, and other animals. We should all be vegetarians, vegans, and new food people. We should feed our family and friends, only garden and farm foods.

Garden and farm foods, have all the vitamins and minerals, that we need. And it's healthy and safe.

We should eat all the variety of food, that is at the store. And we should plant in our gardens, as much fruit and vegetables that we can. We should teach our children, and teach our friends and family, to not eat animals, and to only eat fruit and vegetables and water.

From the time that we are growing to birth, baby, child, teenager, to adult, we should be only eating new garden farm foods. We should never eat animal's, they are wrong and sad, for you to eat. If we can do this, we have really accomplished something nice in our lives. To eat only fruit and vegetables with water, is a nice accomplishment to our lives. This is the nicest information that we could have.

And we should never wear any animal skin leather, feathers, or fur, clothes, because the blood in the skins touch our skins and makes us sick with the Coronavirus. Animals on the outside of our body, as clothes, is wrong and sad to do. Fabric clothes is nice to do.

We should only wear cotton, linen, fleece, velvet and vinyl material fabrics. We should never purchase animal cow skins of leather: shoes, belts, wallets, purses, coats, vests, or pants. We should purchase vinyl and fabric shoes, belts, wallets, purses, coats, vests, pants, skirts, and shirts. We should never purchase any cow leather furniture of: sofas, chairs, and rugs. We should buy fabric sofas or vinyl sofas. We should never purchase cars, that have cow leather seats in them, or motorcycles that have leather on them. We should purchase cars, trucks, and motorcycles that have fabric seats or vinyl seats.

We now have vinyl and fabric, to wear, or sit on. We don't need animals to live with. Let them alone. And be different. Use only fabric of vinyl for clothes, shoes, furniture, and cars.

All schools that teach information of elementary, high school, and collage, should teach classes, about farms and gardens to eat the new foods, that they grow and pick, of fruits and vegetables. They should teach to not eat, drink, wear, or use animals.

Gardens and farms from plants and trees, are ancient, since the beginning of time, and they used to eat only the garden and farm foods, of nature from plants and trees. This is the most safe tradition amongst all. We as the world of people, must change old traditions that involve deathing of animals, eating them, drinking them, wearing them, and using them for items, and start a new tradition in we.

Seems like all holidays in America, involve the false traditions of eating, to celebrate, with a variety of dead animals: on Valentine's day of chocolate with cow milk in it, on Easter of chocolate chicken eggs from cows, and chocolate bunnies, on 4th of July barbequing animals meat from pigs and cows, Thanksgiving of a turkey meat, Christmas of a Turkey meat or pig meat ham, and New Years of Alcohol, and other holidays that involve animals in the food. What are we really celebrating with it all? Death? Dead animal's parts and pieces of their bodies? We shouldn't have animals on our tables, to be with our family. We should be eating only fruits and vegetables, on our tables to be with those holidays, with ourselves, and with our families, and with our city and countries. Let's start a new tradition of this.

Wouldn't it be better to eat and drink from plants, instead of eating and drinking from animals? Yes. Wouldn't it be better to wear plant fabric of cotton, linen, fleece, velvet, and vinyl, instead of cow skins leather, bird feathers, animal fur, and sheep wool? Yes.

The eating, drinking, wearing, and using animal's bodies and fluids, of meat and milk, have been done for thousands of years, and that must be stopped. A new tradition of only fruits and vegetables, must be started for our lives, and for others lives.

We as a world, in our city and families, and individually, need a new pure truthful tradition, of eating only fruits, vegetables, all new, not cooked. Each day can be a new day, of being with a tradition, to eat from the garden and life.

Vegetarian, Vegan, and Fruit and Vegetable People

I have studied foods, and the effects of foods for 40 years. And, in my studies, and experiments, I have found that eating the foods, from the garden and farms, of plants and trees, new, and natural, are the nicest way to eat. I feel the nicest eating fruits and vegetables, instead of eating dead animals, cooked, frozen, canned, or microwaved foods.

Are you on a healthy path this year? Do you want to make a difference, in your life with food? Who ever thought that foods, can make a difference in your life? Vegetarians, Vegans, and New Food People did.

That is who has thought me about it. I was lucky enough to meet a few people, and read books, in my life, who taught me about animals and food.

Those vegetarians, vegans, and fruit and vegetable people, think about food, and the effects of foods. How food affects them. How they feel. And they think about the animals, and how they feel, about what has happened to them. Vegetarians, vegans, and new food people, are kind to the animals. Does the food make them feel healthy or sick? Does the food have meat in it? Does the food have fruit and vegetables in it? Does the food have blood in it? Or does the food have water in it?

This is how vegetarians, vegans and new food people think: "Does the food have meat in it? If that food has meat in it, then I cannot eat it. Does that food have dairy milk products in it? If that food has dairy milk products in it, then I cannot eat it. If the food is only fruits and vegetables, then I can eat it."

As a vegetarian, vegan, and new food person, I have had to change my ways of eating, dressing, and living. Because I took away, the animal meat foods, the animal dairy milk products, I had to give myself some new fruit and vegetables. I had to substitute my old eating habits, to a new way eating habits. And I like it better.

If you are trying to be a vegetarian, vegan or fresh food person or all of them, remember the date that you started to stop eating animal products, and add up the hours, days, weeks, months and years.

If you accidentally ate something you shouldn't, like animal foods, of meat or dairy milk drinks, or milk foods from cows, keep trying. You don't have to start over with the date, you started to be a vegetarian, vegan or a new food person, keep on and keep your commitment to stop eating meat and milk products, and not eat like that again. Keep trying to do better at eating garden and farm foods.

Keep trying to be a vegetarians, vegan or new food person, in your life. Nice things will happen and you will feel better than ever, eating mostly from the garden and farms of new foods. This will be your new way of being and eating each day, and for this year, as a vegetarian, vegan or new food person. Congratulations on not eating animals, and eating only fruits and vegetables all new.

In my life, I have met only a few vegetarians, and a few vegans, in 40 years. And those vegetarians and vegans, taught me what they did, and told me what I could do, like them. So I did what they did, to improve my life, by stopping eating animals, and stopping wearing animal items, of clothes and shoes, and stopping sitting on animal skins leather of cows, of furniture of sofas, chairs, and rugs.

I realized, years later, after I had stopped eating meat, that I was a vegetarian. And then when I met people, who didn't eat all meat of all animals, and didn't drink any dairy milk drinks of animals, and didn't ware any animal leather skins clothes, shoes, or accessories, I learned that, that is called being a vegan. From meeting three vegans, I wondered if I should be vegan? So I asked out loud, in my kitchen to myself, "Should I be Vegan?" and I went vegan.

And then after that, going vegan, a year later, I went juicing and new foods, where I didn't even eat cooked foods, I ate natural, new foods, of the garden, and farms, of plants, and trees.

In talking to my vegetarian and vegan friends, they taught me what I to do, and help me, learn what is better by not eating animal foods, or wearing animal clothes and shoes. So, after being vegetarian and vegan for many years, I went higher than vegetarian and vegan, by being a new food person, not even cooking my foods, eating all new foods of fruits, vegetables, nuts, and wheat.

I learned how to do that, and I can't believe, that people eat animal meat, and drink animal milk drinks, all of their lives. Don't they get it? Don't they realize, what they are doing, eating animals, and drinking animals, and stop? It's nice to do that. I'm happy I learned and believed in that. And, I wish that others will find out about eating fruits and vegetables only, with water and not eating the seeds of fruit or vegetables, and stop eating cooked foods and animal's foods of meat and milk.

Being a vegan or new food person takes work. I have to shop, search, and seek for new foods of fruits and vegetables only, in the food stores, and certain isles, to find all of what I need for the week to eat. I have to find vegan food, at the restaurants that is mostly vegetables and fruit, with no meat or dairy milk in that.

I have to tell my family, what I can eat, and what I cannot eat, when we are together, if they are preparing food for us. I have to really look, over the menus, at the restaurants, to find garden and farm foods, of vegetables and fruit. At the convenient stores I have to look for fruit, raw nuts, vegan granola bars, chips with no cheese or sour cream, and water.

I have to find the fruit and vegetables, that are vegan dishes, made by others, at dinners, without the meat and dairy milk in them. I have to do this alone, because I am the only one where I live, that is mostly vegan, and vegetarian.

I don't mind though, I like being different like that, and I like looking for the food, that I want to eat. I can always find something to eat, that is vegetarian, vegan, or ne food. The nicest of them all, is purchasing food, at the food store new, and eating them at home.

Vegetarians, vegans, and new food people, are leaders and examples, of how to eat for the world of people. They are a small group of people through out the world, yet they have a lead on what to eat. They don't eat animal meat, or drink animal milk drinks. They don't wear animal clothes or animal items. They inspire by example. I like that you are doing that. Keep doing that. They do this in a world that eats mostly cooked foods, and animal meat, and animal milk drinks, so lets be different, and only eat fruits and vegetables.

That Takes Practice

Most people went through life, eating the foods that the family ate, growing up. When I heard what happened to animals, that they made food from animals, I didn't like that, and I stopped eating animals, one by one, over the years, until I completely stopped eating all animals, of meat and dairy milk drinks from cows or other animals. It takes practice to not eat animals. And it takes practice to eat only fruits and vegetables daily.

I had a few mistakes of eating animals, when I didn't know that dairy milk was in the food, because I didn't know about the ingredients. Yet, I keep being in my vegetarian, vegan and new food ways of eating. It has been 40 years, since I have been food conscious, in not eat animal products. I have tired to not eat, meat or dairy milk products of animals, for all of those years on my own.

I had a few people tell me about food, what not to eat, or what not to wear that were animal items. Either I talked to the people in person, or I read the information from a book, I learned from a live presentation, and mostly I learned from me.

What I did was, pick one animal that I ate the least, and I stopped eating that animal meat, for the day. And then I would think about how I feel about that. And then I stopped eating, that animal for a week, until I have a month, and a year and then several years.

After I stopped eating, one animal meat, or dairy milk drink, then I picked the next, animal meat, or dairy milk products, to stop eating, and worked on not eating, that animal for a while. I didn't know I was eating animals, that were made into food, until when I was older. I just thought it was meat or milk food. I didn't know what that was. I didn't think about that. I didn't know to about that. I ate it because my family ate it, a false tradition.

And now, I think about it to better myself, and to stop eating animal foods, and to avoid animal foods at the food store, at parties, and at restaurants.

Since I stopped eating animal foods, and I took that away from me, I then found new fruits and vegetables, that I hadn't eaten before, and I began to eat more garden and farm foods, in my life, and gave that to me, and I like that.

I Tell Them, I don't Eat, Drink, or Ware Animals

As a vegan new food person, I like to talk to others, about what I do, as a healthy eater. I tell everyone. When I meet someone, in person or on the phone, and if they are interested, in hearing me, I know that I only have a few minutes, to share with them, what I do, and how I eat. I usually tell them, "I'm a vegan. Do you know what that is?" I tell them, " I don't eat meat, or milk items. I don't eat animal items, and I don't wear animal leather clothes, or shoes and I don't use that item of leather on sofas, cars, or accessories."

I tell them, "I eat mostly fresh fruits and vegetables." I practice being, a garden and farm eater, instead of an animal eater. I try my best to eat healthy and drink water.

In meeting someone, if I have the chance, I talk about how I eat vegan, and fresh food, and not wear leather, I will tell them. That may be the only time, someone talks to them, about it. And it may make a change for them in their life, I hope. It made a change for me in my life, in meeting vegans. I changed, and did what they did. Some of them tell me, that they didn't know about, what I told them.

I went to a shoe store, to find a vinyl pair of shoes or man made materials, and I asked the lady there if the shoes were vinyl? She had to find out. She didn't even know the difference, between leather and vinyl. So, I had to explain it to her that one is man made, and the other is animal leather made from a cow. I also told her that I am a vegan, and that I don't eat animal meat or dairy milk drinks. She said she was happy, that she knew the difference now.

When you are around people, try to tell them, that you don't eat meat or milk from animals. Tell them that you are a vegetarian, vegan, or new food person, if you want to, and tell them that you only eat fruits and vegetables. Depending on what you are doing with your food eating habit, you may be an example for them to follow.

Maybe you talking to them about the food, may be the only chance that they get to hear, about that someone who doesn't eat that kind of meat, or doesn't drink milk drinks. You may be able to tell them about your eating habits, of not eating meat or dairy milk, and they may find out something from you, and their life will change. Mine changed when someone told me about food made from animals. I didn't like finding out that animals were made into food. So, I stopped eating and drinking animals, as soon as I heard that from them.

What do you say, when people ask you what do you eat? I say that I am a vegetarian since 14. Even when I meet people I always have a conversation that I am a vegan, and I say that I don't eat any meat or drink milk of animals. They might ask me if I eat eggs, and I say no. They usually say, "I don't know that I can do that." They say that they like meat. I tell them that I get sick if I eat meat or milk items of animals.

I tell them that what you do, is pick one animal that you don't eat the least, and stop eating it, for a day, of pig meat. Then try not eating it for two days, then a week, and then a month. After you have practiced not eating meat for a month, then pick the next animal that you don't eat the least of, next cow. No cow meat for a day, then two days, then a week, and then a month.

Do this until you have eventually eliminated, all of the animals, from your food intake. Next stop eating seafood. Then stop eating chicken. Turkey is only once a year, so that is nice to stop. Then stop eating honey, from bees. There you have it, that's all the animals that most people eat. It's much to think about. Could you think about that? And do that?

You have to stop driving to restaurants, that serve only animal meat and milk items, and find new restaurants that serve salads and soups, with no meat or milk in them. Shop in the food stores area only, to buy fruit, vegetables, and nuts. Stay out of the meat area, and cooked food isles.

I know about not eating, drinking, wearing, or using animal's bodies and fluids milks. So, I have a responsibility to teach you and all people about it, so you can accept it, learn from that, and do that. As you learn from this book, about food and animals, you may have the same responsibility to teach people you know, about what you learned, so they can learn from you. We must inform the world of this, to make a change, and help the animals and people. We start with ourselves as an individual, to stop from eating animals, and eat only farm and garden foods new, of fruits and vegetables, nuts and water. Then we tell our family, our schools, our work, our society, our city, our state, our country, and our world, on this our land, our earth, our planet and of our universe. We must inform everyone of this so we can have a new world, of healthy eating habits. We must be an example to ourselves, to the animals, to others, and to the world.

Change in Our Life

We must change the path we eat. We must change from eating animals, to eating garden and farm foods, fruits and vegetables. It's time to change in this world. You might have to do this by yourself, alone, or with your husband or wife, or family, because most people eat animal items, and have no intention in stopping. We must stop eating animals, and start eating fruit, and vegetables, only. The change must first start with you. Change your mind from thinking you have to eat animals. Change your hands from touching animal meat, and animal milk drinks, reach for and touch new foods of fruits and vegetables. Change your body from being a people and animal body, to only a person body. We must change our relationships. Man and woman belong together, so stop having animals in your body, because that is adding animals to your relationship, and that causes problems. The solution is eating only garden and farm foods, from the food stores, to only have fruits and vegetables in your body and in your home. Yes.

Do you have animals inside of your body? Or, do you have garden and farm foods, of fruit and vegetables, in your body? What do you choose? I choose fruit and vegetable body, for the rest of my life. We must create children with a person body. Not with animals in our body, or else the children are being born with will have animal birth defects. Eating animals cause all sicknesses, viruses, and disease. Dis-ease. It is time to change everything around us, if we stop eating animals. Its time to get new kitchen items: the plates, glasses, bowls, forks, knives, and spoons that we used to eat animals with, must be thrown away, and purchase new plates, glasses, bowls, forks, knifes, and spoons, for our plant and tree food of fruits and vegetables with water. This is a new way of being, and is a new change, for the better.

Also get new towels for your new garden and farm body. Change is nice. Embrace it. Change where you shop in the store. Stop shopping in the dead isles. Stop buying dead animal's bodies, and start to only shop in the food department where all the fruit, vegetables, nuts, and vegan foods are, non dairy milks and non dairy cheese, and meatless meats. This is a nice change.

Family Traditions, and World Traditions

Most families grew up and were raised, eating animal meat, and animal milk dairy items, and some fruits and vegetables, both. This is a false tradition. And it should be stopped today. Eating meat and milk, is a false tradition, of the family, and of people in society, at food stores, and at restaurants. At home is where we start, to stop the false tradition, of eating meat and drinking milk. And start eating only garden and farm foods. Start a new tradition. You might be the first to do this. Some people practice eating only fruits, vegetables, and nuts with water, later in life, when they start to meet vegetarians, and vegan people.

I went to as many classes that I could, and read books, about food and learned what to eat and what not to eat, from what people who taught. I mostly learned from myself of being sick from eating animal's milk and animal meat, and stopped that, and started a new path.

Some food traditions are very strong. Like Thanksgiving or Christmas, where they eat turkey. We don't need to do that. A plate of vegetables, and a plate of fruit, will be nice.

Most of the world's population, of families and individuals, have followed the false traditions of eating death. I follow the new traditions, that I am setting, for myself of eating, new foods, of the land and earth, on this planet.

What to Do, About Foods and Animals?

We should stop eating animals of meat bodies, and animal milk fluids drinks. And we should stop wearing animal clothes, using animal leather in furniture, cars, trucks, and accessories as wallets, purses, pillows, blankets, and other items.

The animals were respected at one time, in this world. Animals weren't eaten, in the beginning, and for a while. Yet, at this time, of the world people, have eaten the animals, and used their skins for items. That is wrong and sad. We shouldn't do that because, it makes we sick, and unhealthy, and it is sad for the animals, and it's sad for the environment.

Animals do have rights, they should live and be free, to do what they want to do, without anyone capturing them, and cutting them up. No one, should hurt animals at all. No one, should eat animals at all. And no one, should put animal skins leather, on sofas, chairs and rugs, or in car or truck seats, and motorcycles for seats. We have vinyl and fabric for that now.

We should only be eating, garden and farm foods, to stay healthy, and using fabric and vinyl for our sofas, chairs, cars and accessories. It's not just about eating healthy, it's also about our surrounding environment too, what we live in, and what we wear, and what we have in our house.

We should be aware of what we eat, and what we wear, to make sure we are not eating any animal foods or animal drinks, or not wearing any animal clothes. Why do people take off the skins of cows, and put them on them? I don't know. It's wrong and sad. We don't need to do that, to ourselves or to the animals. We have many other choices to choose from of cotton, linen, fleece, velvet, or vinyl, that is more earth friendly, from the land of plants.

Kitchen Counter

It important to wash your fruit and vegetables before you eat them. Wash your food and dry them off with a paper towel or napkin, is best since others did touch the fruit, in picking it, and at the store to stocking them, and at the check out, to finally get the food to you, to eat.

And it is nice to keep your fruit and vegetables, out on the counter at room temperature, since they grew outside in nature's temperature. I keep my fruit and vegetables, in the bags, on the counter, or not in bags. You must eat them soon, so they stay new. This is how they grew outside, in the fresh air and sun. And you will get to experience eating the food as it grew for you. Keeping the fruit and vegetables in the refrigerator, will preserve them longer, yet they will be cold. That takes away the natural sunlight, that they have been getting all those months they grew, and we need that sunlight for our body. This is healthy for us. Keeping foods on the counter keeps them away from the electricity in the refrigerator. There is no electricity on the counter. And they are in the natural light on the counter, instead of a light in the refrigerator.

Try an experiment with foods that are new, of apples, carrots, and put them on the counter, at nature's temperature. See how long they stay there whole and fresh, they stay in shape and form for weeks.

If you eat animals meat and milk products, put them on the counter at nature's temperature and see what happens to them. They attract bacteria and grow mold. They don't last long. And when they are old they have the Corona virus.

Being sick is what cooked foods or animal items, will do to your body if you eat them. So eat fruit and vegetables new, not old.

Table

I was vacationing in another country on tour, and it was time for lunch. We all went into the dining room where there was a buffet. I filled up my plate with all the fruits, vegetables, and bread that they had there. I was the first one to sit at the table with my food. Soon people started to fill up the seats around me, yet to my sadness I noticed that everyone had piles of meat on their plates. They started to eat all that meat, and I couldn't take it. I felt sick to my stomach to watch them eat meat of animals. So, I got up and walked away from that table of people eating meat, to another empty table and sat down to eat my fruits and vegetables alone.

After the dinner was over a group of people, my friends, came up to me and they all asked me, "Why don't eat meat?" I knew that they must have noticed that I left the table of meat eaters, to sit at a table by myself. So I said to them, "Because I live in the garden and eat there." They didn't say anything, they only listened to me tell them that. People do notice.

Farmers Stores

Some cities have farmer's stores, and they sell fresh foods. You can find all kinds of fruits and vegetables. The farmers, have grown the foods, at their local farm, and then sell the new foods, to the people.

You can walk around and shop outside, at the different tables. You can find out where the food store are, at in the local newspaper, or call the city, to find out where the farmers stores will be located. They are only during the summer months, and usually only on the weekends.

I bought fresh food there before, and I have tried the fruit and vegetables. And it's nice, because they don't sell any animal items, only fruits, vegetables.

Food Journal

You could keep a food journal, for a day, and write down, all the garden and farm foods, that you ate for breakfast, lunch, and dinner. Write down the fruit, vegetables, that you ate, to keep a journal of it. Do this so you can know what food, you have already eaten, and what food, you need to buy for next time. Try every kind of fruit, you can, for breakfast, and try every kind of vegetable for lunch without the seeds. Take the seeds out of the fruits and vegetables, and then eat the fruit and vegetables.

Then you could keep a food journal, for a week, and write down all of the fruits and vegetables, that you have eaten for breakfast, lunch, and dinner.

And then you could write down for a month, what you have eaten for breakfast, lunch and dinner, and a month will be enough to eat all of the different kinds of fruits, vegetables, by shopping at least once a week, to try all of the different kinds of new food, at the food store, from the farms and gardens, of the land and earth.

You could also write down, what kinds of fruit you have eaten in the past. Write down what kinds of vegetables, you have eaten in the past.

Then you could write, about the kinds of meats and dairy milk drinks, that you have eaten, so you can be aware, of what you have eaten, in the past. And write about what kinds of new foods, that you want to eat, for the future.

Write about the cooked foods, that you have eaten in the past also.

Read over your writings, and see what you have eaten, of healthy and not healthy foods. Write about what you want to do today, and for the future of eating healthy.

Food Books

Buy some magazines, that are health informative, either in the food stores, in a book store, or find one on the computer. Then you can read, about food, and how new food helps you.

You could also buy a book, about food, and read about how the food, is there to keep you healthy, and full of energy. I read several books, about food, and learned about a food, that I didn't even know about.

Reading about garden foods, can be very nice for us. We can learn a lot of knowledge from them. Purchase a magazine, or book that is mostly about, new garden foods, and not cooked, or animal items. There are magazines about food, that will teach you about food, and information about it.

Birthday

Everyone has a birthday. And on this day, we should have ourselves, to some special new foods. Drive or walk out to eat, or visit the food store, and buy some special foods and drinks, that you like to eat and drink. Have this with the food stores of how beautiful that is, for you this day.

Instead of eating a cooked cake that has sugar, milk, eggs, or butter in that, make a cake, without eggs, milk, or butter. Vegan. Eat a bowl of fruit. Stay away from the traditional cakes, with dairy products in them. Substitute eggs for olive oil. Use water instead of milk. Use olive oil instead of butter. You don't need animals, in your cake. Could you do this to fix that?

My family took me out to eat, at a buffet for my birthday. And, I usually have the salad plate. They know that I am vegan new food person, so they are thoughtful of me at times.

And for one birthday, my family gave me a fruits, vegetables basket. I was so surprised. It looked so nice. I liked it. I ate it all.

They were thinking of my eating habits, and what I eat, to help me with food.

Life and Death

Before we were born we didn't eat meat or milk of animals. Most people grew up, eating what we shouldn't eat in our days. And when we die, we won't be eating meat, or dairy milk products, or cooked foods. It's not allowed there. I know it. They don't do that there. They don't eat meat, or dairy milk drinks, from cows or goats, in the spirit world heaven of people. They eat spirit food of new fruits, vegetables, with water.

The animals that die are not killed there, nor eaten in the spirit world. The animals are spirits in the spirit world heaven of people, and they don't have bodies because, we at them all away, here on earth. The animals have no body in the spirit world heaven, they are a spirit too, so they are finally free from being eaten again. You can't eat the animal's body in the spirit world heaven, because you at the animal's body on earth, so there is not body for you to eat of animals in the spirit world heaven of people. You must eat new foods in the spirit world heaven, of fruits and vegetables. And, the animals only eat grass, also in the spirit world heaven.

The people are finally free from eating animals, and drinking animals in the spirit world heaven of people. So why wait to die to find out eating animals is not allowed in the spirit world heaven of people. Why eat animals all of your life, and have an animal body? When you could eat garden and farm food, new and feel nicer, have a nicer body and a nicer life. Eating animals and drinking animal's milk and meat is a dead world, because the people mostly eat too much cooked foods, they eat almost all the animal's meat, and they drink animals milks are sleeping and not awake, we need to wake up, and stop that.

I think that eating the wrong and sad foods, is not happening in the spirit world heaven of people, so it shouldn't be happening here on earth. Yet eating meat and dairy has happened here, so we have to not look at it, and not participate in it.

Work on stopping eating the wrong and sad foods, and practice not drinking the wrong and sad milk. And what are the wrong and sad foods? Too much cooked foods, animal meat, and dairy milk items. New foods are the nicest and the best, of the garden produce. Those are the right foods to eat of fruits and vegetables with water.

You won't be eating animal meat, and dairy milk drinks from a cow, or cooked foods when you die, so you might as well not eat them now, while you are alive. Practice looking only at the food stores area of fruits and vegetables of food. Practice purchasing only garden and farm foods. Practice eating only garden and farm foods. It takes practice. It took me years to learn what to do. And I learned it from people I met. I didn't learn in schools, not to eat the animals from teachers, I learned from a friend at school. And I didn't learn to not eat animals from my family. I learned from friends who I met in my life, and I learned from on my own.

We should do the nicest we can, and eat only vegetarian, and vegan, and new food path. And work on our eating habits, this is very important and can really change our life, now while we are living. Don't wait until you die to find out that were only supposto eat fruits and vegetables, and not eat animals bodies flesh meat, or drink animals fluids milk.

Imaging you dead as a spirit, thinking of your body dead lying in the grave, filled with dead animal's meat body parts and pieces, and animal milk, and a few fruits and vegetables. You will get your body back some day after you die, so take care of it now.

When we die our spirit travels to the next life. When an animal dies it's spirit travels to the next life too. Eventually some day you will want your body back. And the animal will want its body back. Yet how will the animals that have been captured, eaten, worn, and used for people, get their body back? Where is the animal grave yard? Where are the animal's bodies? The animal's bodies are in men's and women's bodies, all mixed up in you. And the animals are in the sewers. How are you planning on giving back the animal's body to them? The animals are in parts and pieces of steak, hamburgers, milk, bacon, eggs, honey, cheese, sour cream, whey, ranch, clothes, shoes, wallets, purses, pillows, blankets, cars, trucks, motorcycles, rugs, chairs, sofas, wall mounted plaques, and other items. We will have to cleanse our body of the animals we ate, and we will have to visit the sewers, and wash off the animal's parts and pieces we put there, and give them back to the animals. Yet they don't want that body back, once it has been used by you, they want a new body. Wouldn't you?

If you have eaten dead animal's bodies meat, and drank animal's milk fluids, then you have made your body a grave. You have stolen from the earth of the animal's bodies, that when they die, they are supposed to be on the land and earth, not dead in our people body. Could you not steal the bodies of the animals and not put them into your body? Could you not steal the animal's fluids of milk items, and not put them in your body? Keep them out of your body. They belong to land and earth, not you. You are not a grave, if you eat only garden and farm foods, they will remove the animal's bodies and fluids, out of your grave body, and bring into your body the garden and farms. And the only way to become nature, is to eat it, all fruits vegetables and pure waters.

How are we as a person, husband and wife, family, city, country, as the world of people, going to get all of the animal's bodies and milk fluids back to the animals? The animal wants their body back, like you want your body back one day, after you die and be in the spirit world of death. Again imagine your body is there in the ground filled with all fruits and vegetables, and water, not animals in it. Not mine. My body will be in the grave with fruits and vegetables. No animals in my body of life. I used to have animals in my body, yet I let them be out of me, now they are in the sewers from the animals that I ate before. I feel sad about that. I don't want to die with animals in my body, on my body, or on my items. I want to live animal free. I want to live and die, with garden and farm foods in my body. That makes me happy.

Alone

As I have been practicing being a vegetarian, vegan and new food person, I have lived alone, and I have lived at home with my family. No one in my family is a vegetarian, vegan or new food person like I am. My family does not eat like me.

If my family was in the kitchen, eating meat and dairy milk, I decided to wait to eat, because of that. I have had to wait in another room, until they were done eating, because I didn't want to be in the kitchen, with them eating the foods, that I don't eat of meat and milk drinks, and I don't like to see them eating animals or drinking animals. I don't like to see the animal meat and milk drinks. I don't like to smell the meat cooking. I stay in my room, with the door closed, to keep the steam of the meat out of my room. So I wait until they are done eating, and then I walk into the kitchen, to eat my fruits and vegetables.

It is better that way for me to eat alone, with my vegetarian, vegan and new food habit way of eating. They don't know that I am doing that, so I wait until they are done eating, I don't want to see them eating meat or dairy milk, I don't want to see them cooking meat, I don't want to see the meat, or dairy milk, in the kitchen. I don't want to see animals in the refrigerator, in the cupboards, on the table, or in the sink, or in their mouths.

I don't eat meat or dairy milk, so I don't have that in common with them. They do eat some fruit and vegetables. And they do invite me to eat with them sometimes, if they are eating vegetarian or vegan style, and then I do eat with them, in the kitchen.

So, you might have to eat at a different time, if someone you know is eating meat or dairy milk, to have your own privacy of eating your fruit and vegetables, from the garden and farms.

Fruit and vegetables are individual food items. A whole cow's meat is more of a group, with all of the parts and pieces that are cut up. That is why I am happy living alone like a piece of fruit is alone, yet grows in a group or team. Many people have to eat a cow, one person cannot eat a whole cow. There are many parts and pieces once the cow is cut up. So you're sharing your food with other people instead of eating individual food and singleness of the garden and farms. I eat alone most of the time.

Parents, Children, and Babies

If you have a baby, or small child, buy a juicer, and juice drinks for them, since they can't eat whole foods yet. You could juice carrots for them to drink, for vegetables. You could juice a cantaloupe, for them to drink for fruit. And water is nice for them. Also, vegan milks: almond milk, soy milk, cashew milk, or coconut milk.

Buy a blender and blend fruits together, or vegetables.

Buy a food processor and blend, garden and farm foods, for them to eat. It cuts the fresh food up, into smaller pieces, and they will have an easier time, eating blended foods, instead of whole foods, since they are small children. New food cut up, by the food processor, will be easier to eat. And, it's better than cooked foods, boxed foods, microwaved foods, toaster oven, and jarred foods. They will like it better. And their stomachs will feel better. If they don't like eating whole fruits and vegetables, blending, juicing, spiral slicer, and food processors make the foods easier to eat and drink, and they will like it.

Juicing, blending, spiral slicer, and food processors, make food easier, for children and babies to eat.

My parents and family are nice, yet, now that I'm a new food person, I wish that I could have had my parents who didn't eat animal's meat and drank animal's milk. I wanted to be born to parents who, ate only fruits, vegetables, and nuts, all new. That way I could have had a pure body life of garden and farm foods, of plants and trees only, not a body of death of dead animals that were eaten. I wanted to be raised by vegan parents or fresh food parents. I wish that I had grown up as a child, with a family who all, eats vegan or all new foods only. My family ate salads at every meal, and they ate some fruits, they ate mostly cooked foods, and some animal meat and animal milk drinks. I wanted a family who didn't eat animal meats, or drank animal milk, and ate only garden and farm foods new. Since I didn't have that, and most people don't have that, yet, I can have that with me, now today, and I can have that with my future family.

I wanted to know about this all of my life. If I could do it all over again, I would start from the beginning, of my creation, and be created with fruits, vegetables, and water only eaters, and continue to do so all of my life on earth.

It's important to have babies and children that are eating vegan or new food only. This will help them in their life.

After you blend or juice or spiral slice for your children or for you for a while, then don't keep the juicer and blender and spiral slicer, throw them away, when they are older and can eat solid foods, because we are supposto eat the food solid like on the farm as they grew.

Family and Friends

I tried talking to my family, about them not eating meat, or dairy milk, yet I noticed that they still eat that path, of animal meat and animal milk drinks from cows or other animals. They sometimes purchase for me fruit and vegetables. Yet, I am on my own in our family who eats vegan. Friends, or other people, have listened to me. I have to be careful, in my suggestions, of what I tell them about food, and animals. I have to respect family and friends, if they want to eat meat and drink milk, flesh and fluids of animals. I keep on being a vegan new food person.

I try to tell my family, to eat more fruit, and vegetable, that they will feel nicer, and to stop eating so much chocolate and cookies. After I said that, I saw more fruit on the counter.

My family told me that I need to eat meat. They don't know, that I don't need to eat meat, and that it makes me sick. I need to eat fruit and vegetables, because that is what I like to eat. So I just tell them, that I don't eat that, and I eat fruits and vegetables, and they stop talking about it. Yet sometimes, they say that my food habits have a problem, because I am not eating meat. They don't know that eating meat, and dairy, has made them sick, and tired. They are sick a lot of the time, and they are always tired, and sleep a lot. And, it has made me sick, and tired, that is why I don't eat meat and dairy milk, or dairy food, of animals.

Society has made us think, that we need milk and meat in our eating. We don't need that at all. It is just a false tradition of captured animals, cut up, and then cooked them to eat, when we don't need to do that. We need to eat fruit, vegetables, and cut them up, and drink water, and then we will have, everything that we need. This is how it was in the beginning of time, and this is how it is with vegetarians, vegans, and new food people.

I grew up, eating like my family did, of meat and dairy, because that is what they served. Yet, when I heard, about not eating animals that way, I stopped. And when I got sick from eating animals, I stopped eating animals. Other people taught me and I taught myself. And I ate different from my family with them at meals. I didn't eat the meat that was served, and I didn't drink the milk. I went on my own of eating only salad, fruit, vegetables, and drinking water. I was on my own, to purchase what I wanted to eat, and eat alone with the garden fruit, vegetables, with water.

I wish that my family and I didn't eat animals. I wish that the many people of the world didn't eat animals and wear them. When I realized some sort of food was animals, I didn't want to eat it again. I stopped. I wish that people didn't live their entire life eating animals, drinking animals and wearing animals, or using animals. I don't eat animals any more. I made a few mistakes, yet I keep on eating new foods of fruits and vegetables. I wish they could see, and know to stop eating animals, and wearing animals like me.

We are all spiritual people, as we eat garden and farm foods, of fruits and vegetables and drink water. We are not spiritual people if we eat animal's foods of milk and meat, or wear animal's skins leather clothes and shoes. We are spiritual people if we wear cotton and linen clothes and vinyl and fabric clothes and shoes. Let do this.

Shopping for Food

When I drive to the food store, I get excited to see all of the new food there. All the colors and shapes. I have my favorite foods to eat. I usually buy the same thing every week, and eat the same food every day. I try to buy something that I haven't eaten yet, and experience that. I usually only shop in the food department where the fruits, and vegetables are.

I see the dead animal meats and animal dairy milk drinks, yet I don't get too close to them. I don't push my cart near those isles. I stay away from it. When I do look at it, I feel sad, and I think, "Why? No. Could I not eat those animal's items." I can't believe it. Who wants to eat red blood meat, and white blood fat, that has collapsed veins in the meat? I don't.

I want to eat food that has water in it, from the months of sitting outside in the sun, and on the soil, in the fresh air, and in the rain water. Now the food is ready for us to eat at the store. We get to eat all the fruits and vegetables.

As I shop in the food store, I see others shopping for food. And I notice that that their carts are piled up high with cans, boxes of cooked foods, and animal products. Where are the fruit and vegetables there? They buy for weeks. Food that is preserved, devitalized, and old. I buy fresh food for about a week at a time. At the checkout line, the people in front of me in line, put their dead animal foods on the counter, I see all the eggs, milk, cheese, meat of animals, and I think they are still asleep. I want to tell them I'm a vegan new food person. Yet, I don't. I'm happy and at peace that I know what I know about food. Animals are not food, they are animals. I eat from trees and plants that grow from the land, and I am awake to the garden and farm foods of the land and earth.

The food stores area of all the fruits and vegetables, supply us with all that we need, protein, calcium, minerals, nutrients, fiber, and others. Garden and farm foods are teachers of the earth. They have wisdom and knowledge in them. They were made for us to eat every day all our lives. We need to invest our money in buying only fruits, vegetables, and water for our lives to live forever only.

Isles at the Grocery Food Store

The grocery stores are divided into areas. You have the produce department, with all the new fruits and vegetables.

Then you have the area of the meats of dead animal items. The dairy milk items are in another area. Boxed foods are in one area. And canned foods are in another area. And the frozen foods are in another area. The microwave foods are in another area. Then you have bagged foods in another area.

So I mostly shop in the food store area, of fruits and vegetables. I don't even shop in the meat department, not the dairy milk area. I see it and think so wrong and sad it is. That meat area sometimes smells, if the dead meat of animals gets really old, I noticed, and the food store area of fruit and vegetables doesn't smell. The air is fresh.

I try to shop only in the food store area, of fruits and vegetables, at the food store, to get what I need there as a new food person.

As a vegan and vegetarian I have shopped in other areas, of the grocery food stores, for foods like oatmeal, bagels, vegan soups, canned vegetables or fruit, olive oil, and cookies without eggs in them or milk, olives and potatoe chips with no cheese or milk on them only plain. I usually have to read the ingredients, in those areas.

There are so many food isles of cooked, canned, boxed, and bagged items that really aren't best for us to eat, and its 80% of the food in the store. The produce food of fruits, vegetables and nuts is only 20% of the store.

I like shopping mostly in the fresh food area, because I feel better there shopping. I don't have to read the ingredients. I know that the new foods, are best for me. And I know that I should be shopping in the food store area only, to get what I need for the week of all new foods.

Most of all I like to shop at the food store that only sell fruits, vegetables, water only, they don't sell meat of animals. I like the environment, it is more free and clean to shop at.

What I Eat in a Week

I usually buy the same foods, at the grocery food store every week. As a fresh food person, I buy avocados, tomatoes, spinach, potatos, grapefruit, cantaloupe, grapes, apples, oranges, almonds, and water. As a vegan, sometimes I buy hummus, vegan crackers and mustard, and vegan tomato soup without the milk in it. I purchase these same foods every week. Then I purchase one food produce item, that I haven't eaten before to try it. I get happy of these foods plant and tree based items, because they are my favorite. I mostly shop in the new food store area, I don't usually shop in the other cooked and animal isles. I keep these food items in the bags on the counter. I don't put them in the refrigerator, I like my food at nature's temperature on the counters.

You can copy my food list, for when you drive or walk, to the grocery food store, and try the same for you.

Juicer, Blender, Food Processor, and Spiral Slicer

I found out about juicing, fruit and vegetables, from friends who juiced. So I got interested, and bought a juicer, and a blender. I started to juice fruit and vegetables. I did that for several years. And I was buying mostly foods, that I had to cut up, of fruit like cantaloupe. I usually juiced carrots for vegetables. And I blended almonds for almond milk.

Juicing is a great way to lose weight. It keeps us healthy. I usually juice a few times a week. I like to juice food one at a time. I don't usually mix food in the juicer. After a few years I threw my juicer away, because I realized that it spins the foods in a circle, and food on the farm for months don't spin. So I now eat the food solid.

A spiral slicer is a way to make the vegetables like noodles. They are easier to eat.

Yet, it's important to not juice, blend, and food processor food so much. It's nicest to eat fruits, vegetables, all solid with out machines, like on the farms where they were still and quiet. So we can learn to be still, and sit in the silence of our homes, and be still more in our life.

Blend in a blender
1 orange, and 2 cups of water, blend
1 apple, and 2cups of water, blend
1 grapefruit, and 2cups of water, blend
2 bananas with no seeds, 1 avocado, and 2c water, blend - make sure to take out the seeds of the banana
2 bananas with not seeds, 1 teaspoon cocoa powder (its chocolate without the cow milk, order it on the internet), and 2cups of water, blend
½ c. almonds, and 2 cups of water, blend

Juicer	Food Processor	Spiral Slicer
1 bag of carrots	2 cups of spinach, and 1 tomato- take out the seeds	1 zucchini
1 cantaloupe	durian	1 sweet potato
tomato, carrots, lemon, celery		

Water

Water is the best drink, that we have to drink. It is refreshing and clean. Drinking water right from the sink is nice with a water filter on the sink, or on the counter. Bottled water is nice to take to work for lunch. Keep a bottle of water in the car in case you need it.

Water keeps our mind clear and refreshed. All garden foods are made up of water, all the fruit and vegetables, grew with water and have water in them. Water grows the food on plants and trees. Water is not in meat or dairy milk drinks, blood is in them. Dairy milk is animal fluids from the animal's utters.

If you eat too much cooked foods, or meat and dairy milk, then you are not getting enough water to eat. As you eat fruits and vegetables, then you are getting water to eat in the food.

Try to drink water more than other drinks. Drink water for breakfast, lunch, and dinner, about 1 cup with each meal or not. That is all you need to drink. Unless you feel you need more water to drink at another time. You really only need about one cup of water, at each meal, 3 cups of water a day. Dink one cup of water for breakfast, one cup of water for lunch, and one cup water for dinner. See what is nicest for you.

Water is the best to drink because it is pure. Water is ready to drink, and you can have it from the sink filtered. Bottled water someone else put the water into the bottle and labeled it. There are many words on the bottled water, and sometimes pictures, so pour the water from the bottle into a glass, that has no words on it, to drink it pure. Drinking water at home from a glass is more pure.

If you are not used to drinking water, add lemon or lime. On lemon cut in half, and squeeze it, into the glass with water. Do the same for the lime. Could you buy a case of water at the store or at the fuel station and drink that. Pour the bottled water into a glass, so you don't have to drink the words, on the bottle? Thanks

Could you not drink water from the refrigerator, it has electricity in it from being plugged into the hot outlet and makes the water cold.

Juice is there to drink although someone else made the juice of fruit juice and vegetable juice. They juiced the vegetables and bottled it. The fruit and vegetables have water in them as they grew during the summer months. And the businesses may have added water to the fruit and vegetable drinks. We shouldn't juice our foods we should eat them the solid form as they are, and drank water only.

Could you purchase a water filter for your kitchen sink.

Salad

Salads are nice to eat for lunch or dinner. It's traditional to eat salad dressing on the salad. I mostly ate salad dressings that didn't have milk in them, I did that as a vegetarian and vegan.

Then when I became a new food person, I started using only olive oil on my salad. Later I added lemon sometimes with my olive oil. And after a while I only ate the lettuce plain, without the salad dressing, or olive oil.

I used to eat only oil and vinegar dressing, yet the more pure I ate, the more I noticed, that my stomach sometimes hurt, eating dressing with vinegar in it. I wondered why. I thought that it might be the vinegar, and it upsetting my stomach. Nobody drinks plain vinegar by itself. It's fermented. It's nicest to eat the lettuce plain, to have the flavor of the lettuce. Animals eat grass all day without salad dressings, and so should we eat lettuce plain.

I like the lettuce and the spinach lettuce. So, I just started to eat the leaves alone, without any salad dressings. I eat the spinach plain without dressings.

And then I would have a tomato and take the seeds out of it. I also like to eat a whole avocado, with my lettuce, and tomato.

It is fine to test foods, to see how we feel, and know what is best, for us is to eat, is the new fruits and vegetables with water.

Read the Ingredients

It is very important to read the ingredients on boxes, cans, and bags to make sure, there is no meat or dairy milk of eggs, milk, whey, sour cream, or cheese, in those packaging of foods.

Don't buy whatever is on the shelf, at the grocery food stores, read all of the ingredients. And if you have a question about the ingredients, call them and ask them, about the ingredients. They will be able to talk to you, about that. They usually have a phone number, on the can, box, or bag for you, if you need to call them.

Reading is important, even if the food states that it is fruit, vegetable, or nuts, because there might be dairy milk or meat, hidden in the ingredients, when they don't advertise that there is animal products, on the front of the box, can, or bag, it might be in the back of it.

Some soups are considered healthy vegetable soups, yet they may say, "contains milk". That is cow milk. So buy other soups that don't say contains milk or meat.

Some soups say contains broth, and that is either chicken or cow broth, so don't eat that either it is meat broth.

Some candy has milk, so don't eat that because it is cow milk.

Some orange juice says citric acid in the ingredients, so maybe buy orange juice that doesn't have citric acid in it.

Some pies say contains eggs. The eggs is not in the fruit, it's in the crust. So don't eat the pies that have eggs in them.

There were a few times when I ate something that I thought was vegan, no meat or milk products. I ate croissants, crackers, soup, and candy, that I thought didn't have animals in it. After I ate it I later read the ingredients, and found out they contained milk and eggs. I felt guilty and sad, and realized that as a vegan I ate an animal of cow and chicken. I thought, "No now I have animals in my body. And I have to wait for them to leave me." I didn't eat that food again. And I continued on my way as a vegan. It was a mistake of what I ate so, I started over again, with not eating animal's products in my food. I didn't give up, I kept doing what I thought was right, to eat animal free, and eat plant and tree based foods.

Foods that are in cans with animal items, of meat or milk may have a virus, for being in the can so long, and you don't want to eat the virus, so make sure the can ingredients, don't have meat or milk in them to be safe in your eating habits.

Cooked Foods

As a vegetarian and vegan, if I have eaten cooked foods, I will usually feel a bit sick, and I realize that I shouldn't eat that cooked foods so much, because I have eaten new foods for so much. I am fine eating all new foods. Maybe I ate new foods, all day of fruits and vegetables, and then maybe I ate a cooked meal, at the end of the day, and I got tired and went to sleep too early, and then woke up feeling sick. So I realize that I should have kept eating only new fruits vegetables, as a new food person, and I wouldn't have been sick, and I would have felt better.

I didn't use the microwave growing up, and I didn't have one on my own, yet my family has a microwave and I used it, and I used the oven once for biscuits. And I use stove to steam vegetables, and make spaghetti with sauce, and no meat. I used the microwave to warm up soups and red beans and rice, yet all of those cooking machines gave me electricity, in my body, after eating the food, in the cooking machines. So I try not to use them.

I don't eat the foods, I shouldn't eat, such as overcooked foods, in a pot on the stove, oven, microwaved, and processed foods, and meat and dairy milk products. I try to not eat those foods, that that could affect me negatively. I stop eating foods that made me feel sick, such as garlic, onions, and seeds, beans, and some nuts. And I only eat the foods that make me feel nice and positive of fruits and vegetables, from the land gardens and farms of plants and trees.

At the food stores, they sell animals foods, in boxes, ovens, microwaves, pots on the stove, and toaster ovens, to cook the animal's foods in. Those boxes that the animal's foods are in are miniature coffins, as they have the dead animal's parts and pieces in them, the animals dead bodies are in those boxes and cans. We should not eat boxed or canned animal's foods. They will make you sick, and do wrong and sad things. So could you eat fruits and vegetables, that aren't in boxes or cans? Thanks.

If you were used to eating mostly cooked foods, for breakfast, try something new, and eat only fruit for breakfast like a grapefruit. You are shifting from eating cooked foods, most of your life, now to new foods for your new life. You will be better and you will like it.

You will be able to tell the difference, eating only garden and farm food new, because you can. I think you will like it better, and you will have more strength, and make better decisions in your life. You will begin to attract, what is best for you in your life, and you will meet others who are doing the same as you, and you can share your information about food with them.

In the beginning of time, they ate their foods directly from the plants and trees, they didn't cook their foods, and we should do the same, not eat so much cooked foods if we can, and eat new foods of fruits and vegetables, from the gardens and farms, instead of from pots on the stove, ovens, toaster ovens, and microwaves.

It's nicest to not eat cooked foods so much, eat fruits and vegetables instead. If you have to eat only one meal cooked, and the rest of the meals new foods of fruits and vegetables, through the day.

Eating fruits and vegetables, they will lead out the cooked foods, and the animals meat, and animals milk drinks and animals milk foods. The more fruits and vegetables and water you drink, will lead out the other foods that don't belong there. They will remove the cooked foods and animal's foods from your body, and they will build a new body, of fruits and vegetables and water. That's nice.

Refrigerator

One day I had a realization about the refrigerator. It's plugged into the hot outlet, and that puts electricity and cold air into the foods. The foods are not cold on the gardens and farms, like they are cold in a refrigerator. And there is no electricity on the land and trees, like the refrigerator has electricity in it that gets into the food. And we don't want to eat electricity in our foods.

Then the refrigerator is dark in there, all day and all night, it takes away the natural sunlight's heat that the fruits, vegetables, and nuts absorbed all summer months. Keep fruits and vegetables on the counter, to have the food at nature's temperature.

We might have animal's meat of its body in parts and pieces, of meat as steak, hamburger, ham, chicken, fish, and milk drinks, in our refrigerator, yet we wouldn't have a live cow, chicken, turkey, pig, fish, or sheep in our refrigerator. We could get into trouble for that. So why have their body parts in there? We should only have fruits, vegetables in the refrigerator if we are vegan. If we are fresh food people could we not use refrigerator, and keep the foods on the counters? They are too cold for the foods. They take away the nature's temperature that the food absorbed for all those months. So use counters.

Milk of Cows

I used to drink milk, until I got sick from it. My stomach hurt from drinking milk. I noticed that, so I stopped drinking milk. I didn't like the pain, in my body, from drinking the milk, and I realized I had to drink something else.

I didn't learn that milk, is from a cows body, until years later. So, instead of drinking cow's milk, I found out that I could drink soy milk. I drank soy milk for a while, and put that on my cereal.

Then I found almond milk, coconut milk, and cashew milk, at the food store, years later. I tried all of them. They all taste about the same, and I don't get sick from drinking soy milk, or almond milk.

I realized that I was lactose intolerant, of drinking cow's milk. The soy milk, and nut milk, is much better for me, and for us to drink. It helps us to feel better too.

Drink some soy milk, instead of cow's milk to fix it, and then drink water. You will feel much better. It is better to drink, from the earth, of soy milk, almond milk, coconut milk, or cashew milk, than to drink, from a cow's body, of its milk. Although water is the nicest to drink of all of them.

Cow's milk is white blood fluids from the animal's utters. You don't want to drink white blood fluids called milk from a cow or goat. You want to drink water from the land and earth? Cow's milk, is for its babies to drink, not for humans to drink. It's a false tradition of drinking a cow's milk, that should be stopped. And start drinking from the lands waters.

You can take a handful of almonds, and put them in a blender, with 2 cups of water, and blend. The water turns white, and it looks like milk, with out the cow milk. It is fun to drink, and safe. It is healthier for you and of the earth.

Dairy is: milk, butter, cheese, cottage cheese, sour cream, yogurt, whey powder, ranch, and chocolate. Dairy products are all from animals, cows, and goats.

We should not eat any of those animal liquids milks foods. They are not nice for we, they will make us sick, and unhealthy. Most of our health issues of being sick, and having viruses, is from drinking, all of that animal milk dairy drinks and milk foods. Animal milk has blood in it. Water is nicest to drink.

Meat of Animals

Meat is from animals: cow, chicken, turkey, pig, fish, shrimp, lobster, crab, crawfish, oysters, honey, eggs, and others. It is all from animals and is mostly called meat, and it is wrong and sad to eat. You don't want to eat bloody cows flesh bodies, cut up into parts and pieces called meat. You do want to eat fruits and vegetables, from the plants and trees, of the land and earth.

Eating meat and milk products, is the cause of all our problems of health such as: cancer, ulcers, colds, acne, head aches, hives, stomach aches, boils, blurred vision, loss of hair, loss of hearing, over weight, bowels problems, viruses, and other problems. All sicknesses are from eating animal foods, and animal milks. Garden and farm, plants and tree food of fruits, vegetables makes us healthy, they don't make us sick.

If you stop eating animal food and drink, maybe your sicknesses will lessen, or stop, and leave your body. As you eat only, garden and farm new foods, of fruits and vegetables, with water, you'll be healed, and you won't have those problems. Fruits and vegetables, all fresh don't make us sick, animal meat makes us sick and blind. Blind because we couldn't see the animals, we were eating and drinking, sitting on our sofas, chairs, cars, trucks, and other items.

As the animals were hurt, in the preparation of eating, then you might hurt, in your body, and what they did to the animals, might have happened to you, only because you ate animals. So could you not eat animal products of meat and milk? Could you eat garden and farm foods, that they make of plants and trees, and then nice things that happen to you? You will be smarter, healthier, and happier. And the animals will be happier too. Not eating animals or drinking animals, and eating only fruits and vegetables, is one of the nicest information you could have and experience in your life.

I had a grapefruit and I cut the top off, cut the sides off, cut the bottom off and it looked like a steak. Then I cut the grapefruit in a slice and cut that into pieces and ate it with a fork. That was to fix it from eating meat. I ate the grapefruit like a steak. Then another day I ate the grapefruit peeled.

Some food stores have meatless meat. It looks like meat yet it's not meat. It's a meat substitute made from vegetables. It tastes nice. I like that. Eating that fixed that from eating meat, to eating meatless meat.

Butter of Cows

Here is some vegan information: instead of using butter on food, use dairy free butter, or use olive oil on food. Instead of putting butter on your toast, pour olive oil onto your toast. Olive oil taste nice, and is better for you. Or buy vegan butter dairy free, no cow milk in the butter.

You can use only olive oil, for salad dressing, instead of all the milk based salad dressings, and vinegar dressings that is fermented. Using olive oil, and some lemon taste nice, and is very healthy for you.

Or on your food, you can eat them plain, with no extra flavoring, to see what it is like.

Butter comes from a cow's body utters. And we don't really need it. It's a false tradition that should be stopped. We really don't need anything from a cow.

We need plant food every day, from the land of plants and trees foods, and eat that. After you fix butter with other options, could you stop using butter, and use butter without dairy milk?

Sugar

Could you not to eat processed sugar, in foods or drinks? It is not healthy for you. There is sugar that is called raw sugar, that is better for you. You can use no sugar at all, eat plain when you eat. You can use olive oil, on your oatmeal instead of sugar.

And try to not eat candy, it is very much not healthy for you. Candy has too much sugar in it, and that is not nice for your teeth and mind. Candy bars have sugar in them, and milk in them, that is cow milk. And, we don't need to eat cow milk in our candy. If you do eat candy, find candy that doesn't have cow milk in it.

Coffee and Tea

We should try to not drink coffee. It has caffeine in it and caffeine makes us nervous. It stresses our nerves and makes us sick. And if you drink it late at night, you may be awake all night. It has too much caffeine in it, and that stresses the body, it speeds it up.

We should not drink caffeine teas. They have caffeine in them, and it makes us nervous, and stresses our nerves, and makes us sick.

Herbal tea is fine. A cup of warm tea is nice, before you went to sleep to relax. Try to buy tea that doesn't have caffeine in it.

It's best to drink plain water, daily, through out the day and night. Then after you drink herbal tea, to fix the coffee and caffeine tea, could you stop drinking tea and coffee? And drink water only.

Cooking Alcohol

I don't use any type of cooking alcohol in my foods, because the alcohol is cooked and it changes the food, from new food to cooked food, and it is alcohol based. Even though it says cooking alcohol, I do not use it.

We don't need cooking alcohol. It is unnecessary. Cooking alcohol doesn't have oxygen air in it. Water has oxygen air in it.

Alcohol

It is important to stay sober, all of your life and never drink alcohol. It is not healthy, and it is sad for us. It changes our minds, causes blank outs, where you cannot see, or know what you are doing, it causes car accidents, it causes tickets of DUI, driving while under the influence of alcohol, and you can get that put on your background, and even might have to go to jail, if you get too many DUI's.

Alcohol also causes hallucinations, of seeing what is not there, or hearing what is not there. And it may also cause family and friend problems. It causes too many problems.

The water in alcohol, is cooked out. What is nice for us to drink is water. There is fruit juice or vegetable juice to drink, yet water is the better to drink.

Animals don't drink alcohol and we shouldn't either. We shouldn't go to bars, or parties, where alcohol is served. And try to stay away from restaurants that serve alcohol. Find restaurants that don't serve alcohol.

It's best to be sober.

It is best to be sober from drinking animal milks, it is best to be sober from eating animal's bodies of meat. And be sober from wearing animal's leather skins, feathers, fur, or wool, for your bodies. It is best to be sober from using animals for items or accessories.

Fasting

You might fast, and not have a meal, no food or water, for the day, just to cleanse your body, and mind. If you have eaten too much cooked foods, or animal items, drink some water, and start a fast, where you don't eat food, or drink water for one meal. Simply stop eating, and let your body rest, from having to process all of the food. Sometimes skip breakfast or dinner, and only drink water.

Then you may skip a second meal, and really see how you feel without food. It makes you appreciate food and eating. And it gives your body a chance to rest, from processed food and drinks.

This is a reflective time, to think about what foods are better for us, than what we have been eating, of cooked foods, or animal foods, and animal milk. Eat only life living garden and farm foods, new is nice for we.

You can start a fast, from eating animal meat, and animal milk drinks. Fast from eating animals for a day, and see how you feel. You'll have more energy. You will be more happier. Your stomach won't hurt. Then fast from eating animals for a week and see how you feel. You might like it.

Then you could fast from eating so much cooked foods in microwaves, stoves, and ovens. Eat new foods of fruits and vegetables not cooked.

Fasting from eating food and water, is a way to cleanse the body, of too much food, or the wrong and sad foods. Maybe you skip a meal of food and water to cleanse, or not eat food and drink water, to cleanse for one meal, or for two meals.

Also you may fast from eating cooked foods for a while, for a day, or a week or a month or year to practice eating new garden and farm foods, to cleanse your body and mind.

Fasting from eating cooked foods, will give you more energy with life foods. You will feel better and think better and act better.

Fasting from eating animal products like meat of chicken, cow, turkey, pig, fish, shrimp, lobster, bee, lamb, goat, and other animal's is called meat and dairy milk drinks and milk foods, and we don't need to eat them. Eat fruits and vegetables with water instead.

Meat is the animals flesh body parts and pieces, of the hind part of the cow, or pig. Dairy is from the body of the animals of cows or goats utters of: milk, cheese, sour cream, cottage cheese, yogurt, whey, ranch, and chocolate. It is better to stop eating them all together, and eat fresh garden foods of fruits and vegetables.

We should fast from eating animal meat, and dairy milk animal drinks. If you fasted from eating animal foods, you could stop from eating the confusion the animals suffered. You could stop from eating the pains, that the animals went through, when they were taken to the business of animal's buildings, where they were captured and died of the animals, and cut them up process them into meat and dairy milk drinks and milk foods. That should not be eaten or drank.

The animals shouldn't be dead, and cut up into unrecognizable parts and pieces, of body parts. The animals should be alive, and free to roam and life. Animals have rights, so fast from eating and drinking them, and experience how you feel about that, without them in your body and life.

Overweight

Do you want to know what over weight is? Eating too much cooked foods and animal's foods. When you eat animals they have the tendency to stay in your body longer than fruit or vegetables. Eating animals makes you gain weight and be overweight. And eating too much cooked foods can cause you to gain weight too. If you eat fruit and vegetables new, you tend to have better weight control.

If you want to lose weight, simply stop eating so much cooked foods, animal's meat, and animal dairy milk drinks and milk foods. The weight will leave you away. And could you stop cooking your food so much, purchase new fruit, vegetables, more. And eat them new.

We all must lose weight physically or spiritually. We must lose the weight of cooked foods, animal meat foods, and animal milk drinks, and animal milk foods. We might be over weight, and have to lose a few or much pounds physically, of the cooked foods we ate, or the animals we ate. Or, we may be average weight, and have to lose spiritual weight, of the cooked foods we ate, or the animals we ate.

I purchased a blender and blended one fruit with water. I purchased a juicer and Juice carrots and cantaloupe. And drink that. I purchased a food processor and blend tomatoes, without the seeds, and spinach for salad. The blender, juicer, and food processor cuts the food up into smaller pieces, that is easier to eat and process, and smaller to lose weight, from eating big food of animals like cows or pigs. You will feel much better, and the taste is nice. You won't be overweight. The juiced foods and blended foods will wash away the overweight. Eat small foods of fruits, vegetables and nuts, to be smaller, with water, and you will lose weight. Then after you lose the weight, throw the machines away, and eat the food solid and drink water only.

The biggest foods you should eat are a watermelon, or cantaloupe, all in one day. Not a big cow, meat, steak, or hamburger. Not a big pig, ham, ribs, or hot dog.

Eat as much fruits, vegetables, that you can with plenty of juices and water, and the weight will leave you away, or adjust to an average size. Eating too much cooked foods, and eating animal's meat, and drinking animal's milk, made you gain weight. So now that you know the problem, cooked foods and animals, mostly animals meat and milk, could you stop that, and eat fruit and vegetables with water?

Cooked foods can make us over weight. When I was a vegetarian, and then a vegan, I weighed myself. And later in life, I realized that I weighed more than I should be.

When I became a new food person eating only fruits, vegetables with water, I weighted myself again and I weighed less. I had lost 29 pounds. I thought that was much better. I realized that I lost weight.

I lost that weight, by simply stopped eating so much cooked foods, stopped eating animal meats of steak, hamburgers, pizza, and turkey, fish, and ham, and stopped eating animal dairy milk drinks and animals milk foods of cheese, butter, sour cream, cottage, yogurt, chocolate, whey, and candy. That's all it is that makes us gain weight is the meat, milk, and cooked foods. So if we stop eating that, we will lose all the weight that we want to. I lost weight, and I wasn't even trying to lose weight, that is what I noticed about me. I didn't exercise, I went for walks though, and I ate mostly new fruits, vegetables. Could you eat grapefruit, orange, pear, apple, cantaloupe, spinach, avocado, tomato no seeds, and potato all new, not cooked.

Now if I gain weight, it is because I ate too much cooked foods. So, I stop eating so much cooked foods, and eat new foods, and then I lose the weight again. And then I get back to the weight I want to be at. Eating is all an experiment.

So if you are overweight, like I was of 29 pounds, or by several pounds, 11 pounds, 49 pounds, or even more pounds, stop eating cooked foods, animal meat, animal milk dairy milk, and animal milk foods, and you will lose all the weight that you want, by eating new fruits, vegetables, and water.

When I see someone who is overweight, I think why? "It's only cows, pigs, and cooked foods." The cow is big, and if you eat cow meat or cow milk, from a cow, you will be big too. The body can't process and digest properly, cow meat and milk. It retains the meat and milk of cows and can't leave. So if you want to lose weight and be smaller or average, like a tomato or apple, eat fruits and vegetables only new.

Some people might be big, over weight, extra large, or bigger, and it's because they ate too much cooked foods, and ate too much animal's bodies of meat, and drank too much animal's fluids of milk, and animal's milk foods. A cow is bigger than an apple, and a pig is bigger than a potatoe. Fruits, vegetables, are smaller and cause us to be average weight. So all they have to do is eat fruits, vegetables and nuts, and the cows and pigs will leave their body, and the person will get smaller again. You can do this simply, by eating that apple or potatoe.

Try eating only or mostly new foods of the gardens and farms, of the land and earth, and you will lose all the weight you want, and you will get to the weight you want to be, you will feel better, and you will look better. Even if you are not over weight, you still need to change your body from animal's body, to fruit and vegetable with water body.

You don't even have to exercise, if you don't want to, and stop eating the wrong and sad foods. Naturally, eat the happy right foods, and take a walk at least once a week, or maybe a few times a week, and you will notice the difference in your life, and be happy, and free.

Vegan food, dairy free, without the cow milk, plant based, alternatives to fix them.

Cow milk or Goat milk – drink vegan almond milk, soy milk, and cashew milk, dairy free without the cow milk in that

Cow cheese – eat vegan cheese, dairy free, without the cow milk in that

Cow butter – eat vegan butter, dairy free, without the cow milk in that

Cow ice cream – eat vegan ice cream, dairy free, without the cow milk in that

Cow chocolate –eat vegan chocolate, dairy free, without the cow milk in that

Cow yogurt – eat vegan yogurt, dairy free, without the cow milk in that

Cow sour cream – eat vegan sour cream, dairy free, without the cow milk in that

Cow whip cream – eat vegan whip cream, dairy free, without the cow milk in that

Cow, chicken, turkey, pig, fish meat - eat vegan meatless meat, without the cow meat in that

Chicken mayonnaise – eat vegan mayonnaise, without the eggs

Restaurants

If I drive out to eat as a family, I try to suggest a restaurant that has salad, vegetables, and fruit. And I try to eat sitting in the salad area, instead of sitting in the meat area.

When I look at most menus, they are all filled page after page, of the same animals: cow, chicken, turkey, fish, shrimp, crab, lobster, oysters, and other animals for us to eat. I have to search and really look and read, to find a salad with no cheese, milk in the dressing, or meat in it. I have to tell the server, "No dairy milk, or meat, in my salad. I'm vegan." I sometimes find a potatoe to eat, steamed broccoli, fries, or vegetable soup, this is for vegans.

I saw the food lined up at a buffet, for the people to take the meat and dairy. I don't go over to that area. It is sad to me. They don't know, not to eat that animal meat and animal milk foods. They do have another path, of only fruits and vegetables, like I eat vegetarian, vegan, and new food. I am just happy that I don't eat animal meat, and dairy milk and milk foods, and that I eat fruit and vegetables new.

I feel best knowing that I eat different, from the main group of people in the world. I have to eat different, because now I know that I can eat different. I want to eat different than how the main world eats. And I don't want to have the virus, that is in the animals foods that they serve to the people.

At the restaurants I get my vegetables and fruit and sit at the table. My family usually has meat and dairy to eat and the people around me. I see what they were eating at the restaurant of meat and dairy milk foods, yet I just try to not look at it, and just focus on my salad, vegetables, and fruit.

I also try to drive to restaurants that have mostly vegetarian foods, like salads, vegetables, and fruit.

At fast food restaurants I have tried to find vegetarian and vegan sandwiches, like all vegetables and veggie burgers. I prefer to find a food store and shop mostly in the new food area. As a learning vegetarian, vegan and new food person, this is the best place for you to shop, and eat from, the food store. And eat at home plant based foods, tree based food.

The restaurants appear to be nice, yet they are sad because their menus, are mostly all animals changed as foods. We shouldn't eat their products of animal's bodies meats and animal's fluids milk foods. The table may be set nice, yet it's sad, when they put a plate of dead animals there for you. Could you not eat that? Order salad or vegetable soups and eat that.

The restaurants should not purchase meat of animals, or milk foods of animals to serve to the people. They should only sell and serve fruits, vegetables, and water to the people. Restaurants that do cook animals to eat should be closed, until they can serve only garden and farm foods to the people.

Garden Farm, or Dead Zoo, in Your Body

A zoo is a place where they keep animals to look at. If you eat animals you will have a dead zoo inside of your body, yet you can't see it. How are you making your body, made of garden and farm foods, or a dead zoo of animal's meat and milk? Fruits and vegetables are of the garden and farms. Animal's meat and milk foods are a dead zoo. And which one do you want in your body? What is your body right now? A garden or a dead zoo? At the zoo the animals are life. Yet when you eat all of the different variety of dead animals, you make your body a dead zoo. Sad.

What can you do to change your body, from being a dead zoo, to being a garden and farm body? Eat fruit and vegetables, with water. The farm foods will lead out the dead animals, out of your body. Keep eating new foods only, and the animals foods, will eventually leave your body. It might take years, yet it is worth the wait. Do it now while you are alive, and have a better life. That's something to think about.

I don't feel guilty and sad eating garden and farm foods. I would feel guilty and sad, if I ate an animal's body meat, or drank its fluids milk. Sometimes I feel guilty and sad, if I cook my foods, because I think I should be eating my food new. Don't people feel guilty and sad about capturing many animals, and cutting animals up, to feed it to other people? Aren't they conscious of that? Don't they realized that the food stores isles of dead animal meat, and dairy milk foods, is a dead zoo right there in the store? It's a dead zoo. They just don't have heads, arms, legs, tail or skin and fur any more. How many different animal's, are dead, in your zoo body? How many fruit, vegetables, and nuts are in your garden and farm body?

Garden and farm foods can do living things for you in your life. Dead zoo animal's meat and dairy milk drinks and dairy milk foods, might do dead things to you in your life. We build a home, car, furniture, yet our body is the most important thing we can build in our lives. And have. And our body should be garden and farm, of plants and trees, not a dead zoo of animal's bodies meat and milk.

Animals Pets

If you have an animal, try to feed your pet vegan foods, with out the milk or meat in it. Try to find vegan and vegetarian food, so that your pet is not eating other animal meat products. The animals want to eat vegetarian, vegan, and new food too. You could fix them your food, to eat of the garden and farms. Your pet might like eating veggie burgers, that are made vegan, or other fruits and vegetables.

Elephants, horses, and camels, all eat only natural foods of the earth and water. They are friendly and nice to people. They are usually awake during the day. The animals are friendly because they eat vegetarian. They eat mostly grass, and drink water. They don't eat other animals. So they are nicer to each other animals, and to are nicer to people.

Lions, tigers, and bears, all eat animals and they sleep much. They are not so friendly to people. They get upset easily, and people have to be careful around them, and stay away from them so they won't get hurt. And that is because the animals eat the wrong foods, other animals. They should be eating more vegetarian, vegan, and new foods, and they won't be like that.

So eat only garden and farm foods, and make sure your pets eat garden and farm foods too. I noticed that most animal food all has meat in it. That is sad for them. Animals need to eat fruit and vegetables too.

You might not have a pet, yet if you eat animal meat or drink animal milk dairy products, you have pets inside of your body.

Cut up some grapefruits for the pets to eat, and oranges with apples. And cut up tomatoes with no seeds and potatoes to eat for them. Use a food processor or cut them yourself.

Animals Milk and Animals Meat, Eaters People

Do you know how difficult it is to eat an animal? A steak, hamburger, ham, fish, or chicken is not solid like a whole apple or a whole potatoe. You have to make sure meat and milk doesn't spoil. And it's an animal that was living and breathing. Now it's gone, and in you, and you get sick. Throw up, viruses, and other sicknesses. I don't get sick eating only garden and farm foods of fruits and vegetables.

The animal doesn't want to be killed and eaten. It wants to live peacefully with its family. We should leave the animals alone. We should be vegetarians, vegans, and new food people, who don't eat animals. We should eat more fruit, vegetables, with water.

Most people drive to the store, and purchase animals meat, or drive to a restaurant, and order animal meat, and don't even know that it had a head, arms, legs, and a tail, with fur all over. They don't think about it. Or if they do think about it, they don't care. They want to eat the meat, because they think they like it. It's a false tradition to eat meat and dairy milk. Someone started a wrong and sad example, of eating animals, and many people blindly, copy and eat the animals and drink the animals. We shouldn't do that.

The fruits and vegetables, are here to take back the animals that you ate, drank, wore, and used. The animals are not yours to eat of steak, hamburger, ham, fish, or chicken. They are theirs. And they belong to the land. You cannot eat the animals, you cannot drink the animals. You cannot wear the animals. You cannot use the animals for items. You have to give the animals back to the land. You have to take the animals out of your body, and off of your tables, out of your cupboards, out of the refrigerators, out of the freezers, out of your ovens, out of your stoves in the pots, out of your microwaves, out of the boxes, out of the cans, out of the bags, off of your sofa, chair, and rug, off of your car, truck, or motorcycle, off of your clothes, off of your shoes, out of your house or apartment, out of your office, and out of your stores.

The fruits and vegetables are here to show you, how to do that, in place of animals, use the foods of fruits, vegetables, and water, all fresh, and cotton, vinyl, fleece, and velvet clothes, shoes, and items. This is a new life for you in your home, in the city and society, in the world, on the earth, and of our planet.

The animal used to be alive, yet people have made them into many parts and pieces dead. You don't want to eat meat, or dairy milk foods that have blood in it. It's not nice for you. It makes you sick with viruses. You don't want to make your body, out of all different kinds of dead animals. You want to make your body out of live fruit, vegetables, and nuts with water. That is healthy.

Some people only know hamburgers, steak, hamburger, chocolate candy, milk, bacon, ham, chicken, fish, turkey, and other animal foods. They don't know about vegetarians, vegans, and new food people who don't eat animals, drink animals, wear animals, or use animals for items. We want to help the meat and milk eaters and drinkers, find a solution and a new way, to eat and drink fresh from the gardens and farms, this will solve our problems of animals, to nature.

Someone who eats only fruits, vegetables, and nuts, with water, appears to be people on the outside, and they are farm and garden food filled within their body from the land.

And someone who eats animals appears to be people on the outside, yet in their their body, is full of dead animals meat bodies and animals milk items, so they are people and animal body. If you ate animals of: cow, chicken, turkey, pig, fish, bee honey, crab, lobster, deer, lamb, then you have an animal costume on the inside of your body, put together by eating them, and drinking them, the animals. You can't really tell that people ate animals, except for sicknesses and overweight.

When I was growing up I ate animals sometimes, yet when I realized finally that the meat or milk was animals, I stopped eating and drinking them. Then when I was older I realized that eating an animal, turns them into what you put in the bathroom toilet, then they are sent to the sewers for a while. I didn't like knowing that I changed animals into bathroom toilet waste. They used to be a whole animal, yet they were changed into steak, hamburger, ham, chicken, or fish and sold to people to eat in their bodies, then put into the toilets, and flushed away, to the sewers, to be there for the rest of their lives, in parts and pieces. That is wrong and sad. It should be stopped. Eating fruits, vegetables, and nuts, with water is much better for us, and nicer for the environment of our cities, countries, and world.

The animals are not there for us to eat from, and not to drink from. They are there for their lives to lives, without people doing that to them. Eating animals and drinking animals is a wrong and sad, and should be stopped completely, to stop viruses and all sicknesses.

Eating fruits and vegetables, with water is happy, full of life, and of nature, and you will be happier, and not be sick.

I never bought animal's meat or animal's milk at the store. And I was thinking I would buy meat, milk, cheese, butter, sour cream, and cottage cheese, and eggs, of animals, since I ate that growing up in my family, and throw it away. I'll do that for me, and to save someone else from eating it.

Animals Food and Drink, and Clothes and Shoes, Items

Vegetarians, Vegans and new food, don't eat animal meat, or drink animal milk dairy items. And, some of them don't even wear animal skin leather, or don't sit on leather sofa, chairs, cars, trucks, motorcycles, or ride on animals. Some vegetarians, vegans, new food people have stopped wearing leather. Instead they wear vinyl, all manmade materials, synthetic imitation leather or fabric materials of clothes and shoes.

The synthetic leather and vinyl, is made to look like leather, yet it is not animal leather, it is imitation leather. It is materials from the land and earth, and not made from a cow's body. It is plant, land, and earth items, that they wear instead of the animal items.

When I found out about being a vegan, I threw away my leather coat, wallet, belt, and shoes. I also threw away my feather pillow, and feather bed blanket. I then threw away my leather sofa, and I got all new items. I got a fabric coat, a fabric and vinyl wallet, a vinyl belt, fabric shoes, and a fabric sofa. I got a fabric pillow and blanket. I also got a fabric sofa, to replace the leather and feathers items that I had. I feel better about that. I didn't realize that I was wearing animals, and using animals. I didn't like knowing that, so I changed it.

I didn't realize that I had so many animal products, because of citys stores that were there, yet I did what I could to make a change, in my life, to better myself, and my environment. I didn't want to wear animal items, of clothes on my body ever. So I stopped. And now I have to read the labels, when I buy something to make sure its cotton, linen, fleece, velvet, or vinyl, and not animal skin leather. I want to make sure I life the nicest that I can have while I am here on this earth.

Garden and farm foods are solid foods. Animal's bodies meat made as foods, is parts and pieces. You may eat all of an apple, tomato, in one sitting at the table, yet you cannot eat a whole cow, turkey, pig, fish, lobster, crab, chicken, or other animals because the head, feet, arms, tails, and other body parts were cut off or removed, therefore the animal is not all there that way, yet the animals was made into parts and pieces – this is not wholeness. No one eats all of the cow, as they have removed the head, arms, legs, tail, and skin, this is parts and pieces, that will make a person feeling like parts and pieces. Eating a whole potato, peach, is complete, and will bring life to your body. Eating solid new foods is like a whole apple, makes us one, healthy, and happy. The cow, chicken, turkey, pig, fish, lobster, crab, and other animals are not to eat of their meats and milks in your life.

So as a person is trying to eat better, and learn how to be a vegetarian, vegan, or new food person, you may also learn how to not wear, the animal products, of clothes and shoes, not sit on the leather products of cars, trucks, motorcycles, sofas, and chairs, and not walk on rugs of animal skins and fur, nor use items of feathers down of coats, pillows and comforters. You can be free of all of that, and use fabric materials.

Do you walk, talk, sit, sleep, work, play, think, with fresh fruits and vegetables with water? Or, do you walk, talk, sit, sleep, work, play, think, have relationships, and do other activities with animals meat or animals milk, in your body and spirit?

Eating animal's meat and drinking animal's fluids of milk does nothing for you beneficial. They hurt you. So let's stop that, and start to eat more fruits and vegetables daily, as they do much for us of health and life, to protect you, your family, and your city.

What will we feed the people if not animal's meat of steak, hamburger, beef, chickens, fish, ham, or turkey? Fruits and vegetables, all fresh, with water to drink. What will the people wear and use if not animals skins leather? Cotton and linen clothes, and fabric and vinyl shoes.

Some people have worn leather skins of animals all their life, cows. Some people have eaten meat all of their life, animals. Some people have drank milk all of their life, cows or goats. Some people have driven and sat in automobiles, with cow leather all of their life. So what will they have to do now with no cows or animals, to wear their skins of leather? Some people have dressed like a cow in leather skins, some have dressed like a bird in feathers, some have dressed like an animals in fur, or some have dressed like a sheep in wool from head to foot with hats, shirts, vests, pants, belt, shoes, wallet, and purse. And they sit on cows that are leather skins sofas, chairs, cars, trucks, and motorcycles seats. So, what will they do now with a new life? Eat plants, and wear plants clothes, and drink water.

If anyone tells you in schools, businesses of work, at home or anywhere to eat from plants and trees only, listen to them and do that. If someone tells you to eat animals or drink animals, don't listen to them, and could you not do that?

To eat, drink, wear, and use animals meat bodies and milk fluids products is wrong, sad, lost, disease, injury, empty, dark, illness, virus, tired, sick, confusion, depressing, broken, burden, mistake, suffering, damaging, destruction, lack, danger, disappointment, trouble, dead, parts and pieces, negative, hurt, and problems.

We need to solve the problem of eating animal's meat and milk drinks, and milk foods, with eating fruits and vegetables, and drink water only. Some people don't know that eating animals meat bodies of steak, hamburger, beef, chicken, fish, eggs, honey, turkey, and drinking animals fluids milk, and eating milk foods of cheese, butter, sour cream, cottage cheese, yogurt, whey, ranch, chocolate, and candy is a problem in this world. And it is. So we need the solution of plants and trees foods, for our and for our city and for all the countries, of the world, this will solve them and help us to be free, from eating and drinking animals, to eating fruits and vegetables, and fasting sometimes.

Animals

Animals were not made for us to eat. The animals shouldn't be turned into steak, hamburgers, chicken, turkey, ham, and fish. And the animal's shouldn't eat each other. They too should eat from the land of plants on the earth. We shouldn't eat land animal's, we shouldn't eat air animal's, nor should we eat ocean animal's. They were not made for us to eat. Don't eat anything that has a face, eyes, arms, legs, and a tail. Don't eat anything that goes to the bathroom. Don't eat anything that walks, swims, or flys. It's not healthy. It causes sickness, viruses, and problems. It is wrong and sad to eat an animal and drink an animal. Let the animals alone on the land, in the ocean, and in the air. If we didn't have animals, no one would eat, drink, or wear the animal's bodies skins called leather, not drink milk fluids, or eat meat of animals. We would only be eating plants and trees foods, in the world.

Who started it? Who started thinking that they needed to eat an animal instead of the plants and trees provided for us? Who stood in the field and looked over at a cow and said, "I wanted to eat that cow's body meat and drink that cow's fluids milk." That is wrong and sad thinking. Unnecessary. Life shouldn't be taken from the animal. Life is given to us with the food from plants and trees. There is no life in dead meat and milk products. It's too much work to try to eat an animal, when you can easily eat fruit or vegetables, from a tree or from a plant on the land of the earth. We have to forgive the people who ate and drank a cow first, and forgive everyone else, who does the same. We must forgive our self from eating that way, and start a new way of eating only fruits and vegetables, in our life, in the world.

Animals should not be in our food stores. Animals should not be deathbed, and taken apart and cut up. Animals should not be put into cans, bags, and boxes. Animals should not be in our food store carts. Animal meat and dairy milk should not be in our mouths, animal meat and dairy milk foods should not be in our stomach. Animal shouldn't be flushed in the bathroom. Animals should be more respected and left alone. Some people have animals in their home. Feed them plant and tree foods. Could you not feed them other animals, in their food.

Try to pick one animal that you don't want to eat, and stop eating one animal. Practice not eating that animal. Try it for two days, then a week, then a month, and then a year. And don't drink the animal. And don't wear the animal. You've got to do something different to change your life. Something has to happen to cause you to awaken, to the realization that you don't need to eat animal's bodies meat, or drink an animal's milk fluids to survive. That is not living. Who wants to eat dead animal body meat and milk fluids, all of their life, then die like that? Never having the realization that, they don't have to eat or drink animals. That is sad and wrong.

Fruit doesn't have arms, legs, head, and tail. It has a stem, to collect water until it is ready to eat. It takes one person to eat an apple. It takes about 50 people to eat a whole cow. And they will be sick. The animal is sick, scared, crying, and worried, in fear of its life, before they are dead, cut up, and made into food. Then we ate the animal's meat or animal milk drinks, filled with worry from the cow, filled with sadness from the cow, filled with confusion from the cow, or whatever animal was being captured and eaten. You eat their problems and their problems become yours too. Then we think, "What is wrong with us?" Because you ate the animals, that is what is wrong. Eating fruits, vegetables with water is what is right.

Plant and tree food doesn't have any problems, so eat fruit and vegetables, instead of animal's bodies and fluids.

If the business of animals gave free tours of their buildings, of what they do in there, to the animals, we wouldn't want to see that, we wouldn't want to eat that. We wouldn't want that to happen to the animals, being dead and cut up. We wouldn't want to purchase those items to eat, drink, wear, or use.

You can eat a solid fruit or vegetable and that is life. You can't eat a whole cow. That is death. They have eaten parts and pieces of the cow, that is not oneness. And cows eat grass all day every day, that's how they get protein. So we don't have to eat a cow to get their protein, we can only eat vegetables, that are green to get the protein in our body, like spinach or broccoli.

I was walking and I found a baby bird sitting on the ground not moving. It was behind a car, about ready to back out. The bird couldn't fly away. I detect that the car was about to drive away. So, I picked up the bird, and moved it over to a grassy and leaf area. The bird let me pick it up. Something was wrong with it. It had a problem. I didn't know what though. I tried to comfort the bird, and then I walked away.

A few days later I realized that I took care of a helpless bird, that needed help. I respected nature. I didn't squeeze the bird and make it die. I didn't pluck all the feathers off the bird, and ware them. I didn't eat the bird, like a chicken. I don't eat birds. How did someone get some wrong and sad idea to even do that? It's so much work to puck off every feather, to get the body to eat. It's not healthy. It's not respectful to capture, pick, and eat a bird. We should let them live and fly. Let them alone in nature where they belong, on in our bodies.

Animals don't usually attack people and eat them. So we shouldn't eat animals. Animals usually leave away from people, for safety and protection. People approach animals, yet they shouldn't. Especially not death, eat, or ware them. No animal should be deathed, cut up, eaten and digested out, or worn.

How are we planning to put all of the animals bodies back together again after they have been eaten? The animals want their body back. And if 50 people ate one cow, how are those 50 people planning to gather back, all of the parts and pieces of the cow, to all put it back together again? I don't know. I don't think the animal will want that body back again, after it has been deathed, cut up, eaten and digested and put out in the bathroom toilet, and then last of all, in the sewers. I think all of the animals will want a new body, and not the one that you ate, drank, wore, or used. A dead cow's meat may feed 50 people, and they have to share the animal's body. Yet, an apple, one person may eat it, and they can eat the whole apple and not have to share with other people, they can eat the apple individually.

Animals don't want to be in your men's and women's bodies, or homes, or stores from eating or drinking them: as they are made into steak, hamburger, ham, chicken, turkey, fish, milk, cheese, butter, sour cream, yogurt, cottage cheese, ice cream, chocolate, and candy, and others. All of those foods have animal's meat bodies or milk fluids in them. Could you not do that?

Animals want to live on the land, all of their lives. The animals of cows and goats, they don't want to be milked with a milking machine, for drinks. The animals don't want their bodies cut up into pieces called meat for food. The animal's don't want to be in your kitchen on your table, in your cupboards, in your refrigerator, oven, stove, toaster oven, or microwave, in your homes or in restaurants. The animal's don't want you to eat or drink them. The animal's don't want to be made into leather clothes, and leather shoes for your body. The animal's want you to wear vinyl or fabric clothes and shoes. The animal's don't want to be in your living room, on your leather sofa and leather chair, or fur rug. The animal's don't want to be a leather car or truck seats, or leather motorcycle seats, they don't want you to sit on them. The animal's want to walk on the land. The animal's don't want to be in your bathroom, down the toilet, and in the sewer. The animal's want to live on the land. The animal's don't want people, men and women, to capture them, dead them, eat them, drink them, wear them, use them, or sit on them. The animal's don't want to see themselves that way. The animal's want to be on the land, in the air, or in the ocean. The animal's want you to eat fruit, vegetables and drink water.

It is my idea, that the animals should have not been made. It was a mistake, because people eat, drink, wear, and use the animals. And the animals use the bathroom, on the land, and don't pick it up. That is wrong and sad for the land, and for us. Yet, the animals are on the land, in the air, and in the oceans, and we have to take care of them. If it was only people, of men and women, and nature, here on earth, we would only eat garden and farm foods, of the land from plants and trees. We would have no animals to eat, drink, wear, or use. We don't need animals, or their meat bodies, dairy milk fluids, or foods of milk, or leather cow skins clothes or shoes, to eat, drink, and wear, we need people.

I don't want animals in the business of animals work places. I don't want animals in the food stores. I don't want animals in my house. I don't want animals in my kitchen. I don't want animals in my toilet. I don't want animals in the sewer. I don't want animal's leather or fur on my furniture of sofas, chairs, or rugs. I don't want animal's leather in my car. I don't want animals in my mouth. I don't want animals in my stomach. I don't want animals in my body. I don't want animals for my clothes or shoes. Yet we have to have them here, because they are here, yet not for us to eat, drink, wear or use.

All viruses are caused from eating animals, or drinking animals, and breathing in the air, from the cooked animals on the stove, or ovens and barbeques in our city, and at home. All sicknesses and viruses are caused by eating and drinking animals. So could you stop doing that, and the virus will leave your body, and you will be back to health again?

We should have pictures of a cow, chicken, turkey, pig, fish, at the stores by the meat and milk to show people, what the foods are. If people could see a picture of the animals, then we might not eat them. We have to find the animals we ate that are called steak, hamburger, beef, ham, roast, hot dog, turkey, fish, salmon, shrimp, crab, lobster, and lamb. We have to find the missing animals that we ate, and give their bodies back to them. Could we stop purchasing animals to eat, and purchase fruits and vegetables with water? Thanks

Nature put the animals on the land, in the air, and in the ocean. Man put animals in their body, and on their body, and on their items, and that is against nature. We must forget, stop, and let alone animals making them die, eating them, drinking them, wearing them, and using them.

How are we planning to stop it? Eat fruit and vegetables, and use cotton, linen, fleece, velvet, and vinyl clothes and shoes, and items every day for all of our lives. This will fix and solve our problems with solutions. This will be better for us, and for our countries, and for our world, and for our planet, of the universe. Something new.

Hunters of Animals, and Business of Animals

As I was on the computer, I found an internet page that has videos, of slaughter houses, with animals being dead and cut up of: cows, chickens, pigs, and sheeps. I watched all of the animal videos. I didn't know that they dead the animals, cut them up for food, and skinned them to make clothes, and shoes, and items. It was very wrong and sad. I don't know how those people do that. I couldn't do that. It was very informative. I didn't like what they did to the animals. I think that the animals don't want to walk into the Business of Animals Building. I call their place of work, Office of People and Animals, slaughter buildings, or Business of Animals, not slaughter houses because it is a building, not a home. The slaughter home, is their homes, with all the animal leather skins, furniture of sofas, chairs, lamps, rugs, trash cans, cars, trucks, and other items are.

The people were stealing animals, from the land, where they belong for the past 2000 years. This has been a dark secret of selling animals for food and drinks, meat and milk, instead of fruits, vegetables and water. They have had to name the animal's bodies and fluids of milk and meat that, because if they called it animal's food of cows, chickens, pigs, turkey, fish, or other animal's, we wouldn't eat them. Stealing the bodies of animal's flesh meat, and stealing the fluids of animal's fluids milk, to eat and drink.

Stealing the animal's skins, called leather, for clothes, shoes, furniture, automobiles seats, and other items. Stealing animals is a sin, that should be stopped. They people should only produce fruit, vegetables and water, to eat, drink and use for items, or they should have furniture stores that sell cotton sofas, chairs, and rugs for the people's homes in the world in our citys. This is much better and nice.

Could you throw away all animals leather cow skins items, and purchase fabric sofas, chairs, rugs, bed blankets, trash cans, lamps, car, truck, and other items to fix it and have a new home. Yes.

So sometimes I watch videos on the computer, of fruit trees and farms, of the people picking fruit and vegetables, and packaging them for sale for the people in our city. Much nicer.

The office of people and animals, should have tours of the slaughter buildings, or business of animals, to see what happens in there, to elementary schools, high schools, colleges, work businesses, and homes, so they can see and experience what is done there. They wouldn't like it. It's wrong and sad. $10 tickets for adults and $5 tickets for children to see what they did there to inform them. then close the building and take it down and throw it away.

It's much easier to tour a farm or garden, and pick and apple and eat it. That's happy and kind.

It's a burden on the people to hunt, and death the animals, it's a burden on the people to cut up the animals into parts and pieces, it's a burden to sell animal's meat, and milk items, to the people, it's a burden to eat, drink, wear, and use dead animals.

I realized the if we eat animals, drink animals, or wear animals, then the hunters who hunt animals of the air, ocean, and land catch them and sell them for food and clothes, the manufactures of animal meat and animal milk drinks, and the food stores and restaurants, they all own the animals, and they shouldn't. They control the animals, and then if you eat the animals, then the animals control you, your body, and your buying food with your money. They are in it to make money, yet it is the wrong and sad work business. They started the viruses and sicknesses, then the people had that sickness from their animal foods and animal drinks that they ate and drank.

Because they have animal businesses of hunting, and manufacturing animals, doesn't meant that we have to participate in purchasing, eating, drinking, wearing, or using the animal foods and drinks that they catch, dead, cut up, produce, and sell. They are not feeding you new foods, they are feeding you animals, and animals are not food for us to eat. They should be farmers and produce fruits and vegetables, and water, or have a furniture stores. That would be much better for all people, and for the environment and society of the world.

Animals have it more sad than people. Animals are hunted on the land, air, and oceans. Animals are put into prison slaughter buildings, and are dead, and cut up, by being cut up into parts and pieces, eaten, drank, worn, and made for items. Animals have a wrong and sad life in that building, in our stores, and in our bodies, then out of our bodies. The business of animals cut off their head, arms, legs, and tails, and take off their skins and fur, feathers, or wool. Then they cut them up, and sell all of their separated body parts, to the people to eat, drink, wear, or use. When you eat a steak or chocolate candy bar, you don't see the head of the cow, you don't see the arms and legs of the cow, you don't see the tail of the cow. You only see the changed animal body parts, and pieces of the animals. What hope do we have for the animals? What hope do we have for the people, who eat animals and drink animals? Start with you and stop that for yourself first, then tell others. Animals are slaves to people, if we dead them or cut them up, and eat them and drink them. It's wrong and sad. And the people are slaves to eating and drinking animals, that should be stopped, and be free eating fruits and vegetables with water.

It is wrong and sad to hurt people. So, why isn't it wrong and sad to hurt animals of the air, land, and ocean? We should have a law that doesn't let people capture animals, dead animals, eat animals, drink animals, wear animals and use animals on items. We don't do that to people, so we shouldn't do that to animals? Could you stop hunting animals and capturing them? Could you stop cutting up the animals and taking them apart, cutting up animals? Could you stop selling animals to people to eat, drink, wear and use? Could you leave that old world away, and find a new world? Find new work to do that doesn't involve animals. Animals are not ours, animals belong to nature, and to the land. Could you free the animals? Could you free yourself?

Hunters, business of animals, stores, restaurants, have changed our world of light and life, to a world of darkness and death, by capturing the animals, cutting them up, and selling them for food. They are denying nature, they are denying gardens and farms, they are denying fruits, vegetables, and water. Farmers accept nature, farms, gardens, trees and plants of fruits, vegetables, and water. That's nice.

The hunters and business of animals have changed our minds, for us into thinking we need animals to eat, drink, wear, and use in our lives to survive. Someone had the wrong and sad idea, to do that to animals, to eat and drink animals, and passed it along to others. They changed our minds and eating habits, for us into thinking we need animals bodies flesh, cut up parts and pieces, to eat called meat. And they changed our eating and drinking, for us into thinking, we need animal's body white blood fluids to drink. They also changed our minds from wearing clothes from plants materials fabric of cotton, for us into thinking we need animal's skins, called leather to wear for clothes and shoes, use for items, furniture and vehicles. We were cow men and cow women, instead of nature men and nature women only. Now almost all the world is doing it. And could it be stopped? And something new started?

The hunters must stop hunting and capturing, the animals alive or dead. The hunters must stop selling the animals, to the business of animals. The businesses of animals must stop, dead the animals, cutting them up, and selling them to stores of grocery food stores, restaurants, clothing store, shoe stores, automobile stores, and other items stores. So what could they do, if they don't dead, cut up, and sell that to the people? They can be farmers of food, clothing, furniture, and other items. That would be nicer for our homes, cities, and the world.

And a new world must be, of the farmers foods, from the gardens and farms. The businesses of hunters and business of animals have caused men and women, to put the animals, that were on the land and earth with their families, in boxes, cans, jars, pots on stoves, ovens, refrigerators, freezers, cabinets, tables, plates, glasses, stomachs, in plastic bags, paper bags, in wrappers, saran wrap, ground to a pulp or powder, in the microwaves, in the refrigerators, in freezers, in the cupboards, in their bodies, on their bodies, in their vehicles, in the toilet, and in the sewers. Yet, the only food that should be put in our body, kitchen, or items is the garden and farm foods only from nature of the land and earths, of fruits and vegetables with water.

We don't need hunters and business of animals to do that on this earth, land, citys, homes, world or in our stores and restaurants. We need farmers who plant, grow, and pick fresh foods. Could you not purchase hunters animals of the land, air, and ocean? Could you not purchase business of animal's meat, dairy milk drinks and dairy milk foods, clothes, shoes, cars, motorcycles, rugs, chairs, sofas, and other items of animals? Hunters and slaughter buildings and stores and restaurants that all hunt, cut up, sell animals are all against nature, against the land, against the earth, and against our planet. Could we stop that? We must close those buildings that do that to the animals, and plant more fruits and vegetables.

If you eat animal's bodies and fluids, of meat and milk drinks, then you are wrong and sad to the hunters and business of animals, and what they do there. They take apart the animals. They are making people sick with sickness and viruses, by getting them to eat animals, drink animals, wear animals and use animals for items. The hunters and business of animals are wrong and sad to capturing animals, dead animals, and cutting up animals, and selling animals to the people of the world. They are battling and fighting the animals, it's a war between people, and animals. And the animals are losing. Don't let the hunters and business of animals and stores, that sell animals, win, by not buying their food of meat, milk items, clothes, and leather sofas, chairs, rugs, motorcycles, cars, and accessories and items. It's wrong and sad. So, be happy and let the farmers help you, with new foods of nature, from plants and trees, of the land and earth.

The animals are crying and worrying, have anxiety, stress, pain, and fear of people that dead, cut up and eat, drink, wear and use them. then we eat that worry anxiety, stress, pain, and fear in the meat and milk of animals. When we eat meat or milk items of animals, we have the animal's problems, and their virus is given to us, then we have the animal's viruses. We need to, and have to, save the animal's from the hunters, business of animals, and stores that do that to them. We need to rescue the animals by leaving them alone, on the land. We need to rescue the animals by not eating, drinking, wearing, or using them for items.

It's a secret that animals were made into foods. If we knew that the meat and milk drinks and foods were animals, we wouldn't eat that. We need to find out about the past history, of what people did, to the animals of capturing them, deathing them, cutting the animals up for food and drinks, so we won't eat and drink animals. It's better to eat fruits and vegetables and drink water, for all of our lives.

Warning, danger, caution, and problems: don't eat animal's bodies of meat and milk fluids, or wear animals leather skins, feathers, fur, or wool, that were hunted, made in business of animals, and sold to stores. They will make you sick of your body, and of your life of what you do. Attention, solve, and solutions:

eat, drink, wear, use natures land gardens, and farms foods of the earth. Use cotton, vinyl, linen, fleece and velvet, clothes and accessories. It will be better for us in our lifes, on earth of the land in our cities and homes.

Our world needs help with the people in what we eat, drink, wear and use. Our world needs help with the animals to not be captured, dead, cut up into parts and pieces, and sold to the people. They need to be free on the land. We all must help. Eating an animal is the end of that world, because there are no seeds to plant in an animal's body of meat or milk, to grow food or drink. The start of the world, is eating fruits and vegetables that have seeds, to plant and grow more food, and that is the start of a new world. Vegetarians, vegan, and new food people don't eat animal's, they eat new foods of the land and earth, from plants and trees.

How will we feed and clothe all of the people, if we stop hunters from hunting animals, close down all of the business of animals who take apart animals, stores who sell animals products, to wear and use, and restaurants that serve animals to eat? There won't be enough farm and garden foods, to eat and fabrics to wear, and use right now. So, we need to plant more trees, plants, gardens, and farms to supply us with that for all the people, to have a new life of nature plant items, instead of using animal bodies foods, or using animals fluids to drink.

If we can stop the hunters from hunting dead and stealing the animals, and the business of animals from hurting, taking apart, cutting up, and selling the animals for food, drinks and making animals clothes and items, restaurants from serving animals for food and drinks, and stores from selling clothing, shoes and items made from animals, our world would be a better place for the people. They all are breaking the law of nature, they are breaking the law of the land, they are against nature and against the land. Everyone should be living man and living woman, the animals should be living, as the earth is living of nature's trees and plants, and of the land, by eating fruits and vegetables and water. Not cooked foods, or animal's foods and animal's drinks.

Could you take your buildings of animals, down to the ground, and throw the building away? And plant grass there with two trees where the building was? Could you find new work to do like be a farmer? Have a fruit store of farm fruits trees for foods of grapefruit, orange, apple, pear, almond nut trees or peanuts, or plants of avocado, tomato, potato, spinach, or cantaloupe? Or, could you have a furniture store of sofas, chairs, and rugs of fabric of cotton, linen, fleece, velvet or vinyl materials for clothes, shoes, sofa and chair seats, cars seats, or truck seats?

Farmers are careful with the new foods for us. And we should be nice to our foods. And eat nice foods new foods of the plants and trees of the land and earth. Were in America where it is the land of the free, yet the animals are not free, in the buildings of animals, if we death them and cut them up for food and drinks. Let's let the animals be free, and let's let us be free by not eating or drinking animals in America and other countries.

The owners of the hunters, slaughter buildings, business of animals, now were sent here to earth to stop, the family traditions of capturing the animals, deathing the animals, and cutting the animals, up for food and drinks. If you are strong enough could you stop the family tradition, and close your old business of animals, and open a fruit store and sell fruits, vegetables, and water, or open a furniture store, and sell food or fabric furniture, sofas, chairs, and rugs? That would be nice for you, for we, for the animals, for the world. You were sent here to wake up, and take off the blinders, from your eyes, to see the light of nature, instead of seeing the darkness of animals work. Work with nature, not animals. This is nice.

I have been traumatized by what has been happening, in the world of people, and animals of capturing them, deathing them, cutting them up for food meat, and drink milk, and cow skin leather, clothes and shoes, and other items. It's sad to wake up to this realization. And I'm happy to wake up and realize, what could be done to stop it, and start something new, of fruits, vegetables and water, and fabric clothes, shoes, furniture, and other items, for our lives for our world. Thank you.

How to Eat Food

I peel a grape fruit of its skin, and eat the food of the grapefruit. I eat the apple or cut the apple and eat it with a fork. I cut the tomato, take out the seeds, and eat the tomato with a fork. I cut the potato with a knife and eat it with a fork new, not cooked. I cut the cantaloupe with a knife in half, cut the half into slices, then cut out the food into pieces and eat that. I use a white cutting board and then put the fruit or vegetable on my plate. I used to eat an apple by biting it, not I cut the apple with a knife and eat it with a fork. It's much nicer that way.

We should eat our food new not cooked, that is old. If we eat our food new we have a higher life and sense and feel better. We are healthier. There is a spiritual high you can sense in your mind and body if you eat the fruits and vegetables new, not old.

We shouldn't eat so much cooked foods, or none at all eventually. For a day eat all new foods to see how you sense better. Thanks.

Without the Seeds

It is best to cut out the seeds from fruits and vegetables. I cut out the seeds from bananas and tomatos. I used to eat the seeds of foods, and then I learned from someone to not eat the seeds. Because, seeds grow outside in the ground, and we should plant the seeds in the ground. If we eat seeds they grow spiritually in we. Eat only the food and not the seeds. It takes time to cut the seeds out of foods, yet it is worth the time to do that.

If you've eaten animals of cows, chickens, turkey, pig, fish or other animals they do not have seeds to plant in them. A steak, hamburger, meat, chicken, ham, bolony, hot dog, ribs, cheese, milk, eggs, honey, sour cream, cottage cheese, whey, chocolate and ranch don't have seeds in them of the animals meat and animals milk foods. And since the animal's foods don't have seeds in them, you don't have anything to plant to grow a plant or to grow a tree to receive food from them. So eat fruit and vegetables and take out the seeds and plant them to have more foods.

Animals don't have food in their bodies. They don't have seeds in them to grow food. So could we not eat animals meat and not drink animals milk? Fruits and vegetables have food in them and water, so could we eat fruits and vegetables? Fruits and vegetables have seeds in them to plant in the ground outside in the yard or on a farm. Could you cut out the seeds and not eat any seeds, like cut out the tomato and banana seeds? Thanks.

Its important to remember that in a seed of fruits and vegetables is a tree with many fruits on it, or a plant with vegetable on it.

Wheat

Could you purchase new wheat at the health food store? They are wheat grains that you could soak 1 cup of wheat and 2 cups of water

over night, and then they are ready to eat new the next day for lunch. This fixes the bread from eating bread cooked, to eating wheat new.

Dream

One night I had a dream that I was sitting at the table with my family. We were having dinner. The table was set and meat was on the plates. I stood up and said, "I cannot partake of this meat of animals." And I walked away from the table. That was my dream. Even in my sleep I would not eat the animal meat. I should have went and got some fruit and vegetables and ate that. I usually do.

Two Lifes, in One World

If you have the chance to be born to vegan new food people who eat only fruits and vegetables and drink water, take it. We could grow up eating only fruits and vegetables, and wear only cotton or linen clothes and vinyl and fabric shoes. Live a life of nature free of the land and earth, this is one life. This is the solution to solve our lives and live happy and free of nature.

The other life was being born to parents who ate animal's meat bodies and drank animal's cow milk dairy items, and wore animal's cow skins leather clothes and shoes. This is the problem of eating animals and drinking animals and wearing animals and living an animal's life. Could we stop this and start to live the other life of nature?

We only have one life to live on earth so let's make it a life of nature with fruits and vegetables and water.

See the Future on Earth

We as a people must see ahead of the future of our world on earth. We must hold a space and place for a world to be functioning, living and surviving on fruits, vegetables, and water only. No dead animal eating meat, and no dead animal drinking milk. We must have this vision in our eyes, in our minds and in our body, a free nation of life foods for the world. For every person to live by and to eat by individually, as a couple married, and as a family of parents and children, garden and farm foods new, not cooked so much more new, and no animal items for foods.

We must look at the next year, where will you be in your eating habits? Where will the world be in a year? Where will the world be in five years with that's eating habits? And ten years, 100 years, and 1000 years? We must be done with eating death, animals, and we must be in alignment with life foods for our future. We can't keep going on eating dead things, we must eat life things foods. We must be here on earth and eat right new foods of fruits and vegetables with water every day. And do this for all of our lifes. And teach our children to eat life foods, and they will teach their children to eat life foods too.

We must disassemble the animal's foods world, we must take it down and stop it completely. We can't keep going on and on deathing animals and cutting up animals and eating animals, drinking animals and wearing animals. We must convert and change to farm land of trees and plant foods based. We must hold this vision and see a clean world. It's time for a change in this world, and the change starts with you. With me. With we. We must separate ourselves from the dead food of animal's bodies and fluids, to a world of solid fruit and vegetables on a daily basis. Food from the trees of life, and plants of life.

We must prepare for our future worlds, eating system of life living foods for everyone, every day, all day, today and tomorrow and forever on earth. We must have a world of living life of people eating fruits, vegetables and drinking water. The choice is yours to choose life foods new for today and for your future with your mate together, a sacred union and spiritual with garden and farm foods, this is our inheritance for our bodies for our lifes, to live in the land of the living on our planet in our universe.

Some of the foods we should take with us into the future is grapefruit, oranges, apples, cantaloupe, lemons, bananas, spinach, tomatos, potatos, peppers, avocados, and other foods. We should not take meat or milk with us into our future.

Book Review

To keep is simple, be with who you are supposed to be with, wait for them to be in your life. Him and Her. Eat fruits and vegetables without the seeds, and drink water. And eat new foods together for all of your lifes. Don't eat so much cooked foods, maybe a veggie burger, or vegan grilled cheese sandwich, with dairy free cheese, and dairy free butter. Don't eat animal's meat bodies, or drink animal's milk fluids. And don't wear animal's cow skins leather clothes, shoes, furniture leather seats, or automobiles leather seats. Trade the car in for fabric seats, and throw the furniture away, and buy fabric furniture. Throw the leather, feather, fur, and wool clothes away and buy fabric clothes of cotton, linen, velvet, fleece, and vinyl and fabric shoes. This will heal you and make your life better. If you have the money build a metal framed house. Metal is living and alive material, not dead like a tree once you cut the roots off, and cut the branches off, it's a dead tree. A metal house is nicer, with cement walls painted white all one, and cement roof painted white all one. Not brick or tiles, they are like puzzle pieces, too many pieces. Remember to keep it simple.

Could We Eat Fruit and Vegetables, not eat so much cooked foods, and not eat animal's milk and meat, Information

Sharon Jacobs

All Types of People Concerning Food:
Fruit, Vegetable, Water People

People who eats only, new foods of the garden and farms, of the land and earth, of plants and trees:
New fruits
New vegetables
New water
New food people don't eat cooked foods.
They don't eat animal meat, drink animal milk, or eat any milk dairy food: cheese, butter, sour cream, cottage cheese, eggs, or honey.
They don't ware animal cow skin leather: pants, skirts, shirts, vests, coats, shoes, wallets, purses, they use vinyl or fabric items.
They don't sit on animal cow skin leather: sofas, or chairs, they use vinyl or fabric, sofas and chairs.
They don't drive in animal cow skin leather: cars, trucks, or motorcycles seats, they use vinyl, or fabric cars seats.
They like to teach others how to be a New Food Person, of the garden and farms, of plants and trees for food.
New Food, garden food, farm food, is the most pure of all nature and the nicest decisions to eat, in life.

Blending, Juicing, and Food Processor People

People who blends or juices, with a blender or juicer, the fruit or vegetables, making sold form food, into liquid to drink.
They drink the fruit and vegetables, instead of eating the food, in solid form.
A food processor cuts the fruit and vegetables, up into smaller pieces so it is easier to chew and eat.

Vegan People

People who don't eat any meat of animals at all.
They don't drink, or eat, any cow milk dairy fluids of: milk, cheese, butter, sour cream, cottage cheese, whey, chocolate, ranch, eggs, or honey.
They do eat some cooked foods, without any dead animal meat, or cow dairy milk in it.
Vegans don't ware any animal cow skin leather from cows, they only ware fabric clothes.
They don't drive in cow skin leather cars, trucks, or motorcycles seats, they only drive in fabric or vinyl cars seats.
They don't sit on cow skin leather furniture of sofas and chairs, they only have vinyl or fabric furniture.
They don't walk on animals skins rugs.
They like to teach others, how to be a Vegan.

Vegetarian People

People who don't eat some meat, or some dairy of animals, they are just starting, to stop eating animals.
They eat cooked foods, without meat, not in the food. Just starting the learning of being a vegetarian.

Cooked Food People

People who cook and eat fruits and vegetables, from cans, and cooks them in a pot on the stove, oven, toaster oven, and microwave.

Animal Milk and Animal Meat People

A person who eats, animal's bodies meat and drinks the milk fluids of cows, or goats, and eats cow milk dairy foods of: butter,
cheese, yogurt, ice cream, whey, ranch, chocolate, eggs, or honey, and they eat the meat of animal's bodies.

Could we live in the solution, instead of in the problem? What is the problem? Eating, Drinking, and Wearing Animals.

What is the solution? Eat new food of fruits and vegetables, and water.
Could we stop eating and drinking animal milk, and meat items, and eat garden and farm foods, of fruit and vegetables?
Could we stop cooking our foods? Cooking takes out the vitamins and minerals. Could we eat the food new of fruits and vegetables?

Could We Eat All New Foods, from the Gardens, Farms, Fields, of Plants and Trees? Fruit – all fresh

Grapefruit
Grapes
Peaches
Plums
Pears
Apples
Blackberries, Blueberries
Raspberries, Cherries
Watermelon
Cantaloupe
Oranges
Banana

Vegetables – all Fresh

Lettuce, Spinach, Basil
Potato, Red Potato
Zucchini, Yellow Squash
Red Pepper, Green Pepper,
Tomato Red and Tomato Yellow
Carrots
Cauliflower, Hiccima

Avocado, Brussels Sprouts,
Celery
Black Olives
Cabbage
Lemon, Lime

Nuts –not roasted, or salted, fresh

Almonds, Peanuts, Cashews, Pecans, Walnuts

Water - from the kitchen sink filtered, or bottled water.
Could we eat the food new, and not cooked, steamed, canned, blended, juiced, dried, or cut up by the store?
Could we eat all plant new food, purchase land, plant gardens and farms, plant fruit trees, and sell new food?
New Fruits and vegetables.

Could We Stop Eating All Animals bodies meat?

cow, chicken, pig, fish, turkey, bee honey, shrimp, crab, lobster, oyster, lamb, deer, and other animals

Could We Stop Drinking, Eating, Animal Milk Dairy Drinks and Food?

milk – from a cow
butter or margarine - from a cow
cheese – from a cow
sour cream - from a cow
cottage cheese - from a cow
yogurt - from a cow
ice cream – from a cow
chocolate – from a cow
whey– from a cow
ranch – from a cow
Goat – milk from a goat

Could We Stop Eating Dead Animal Meat from their bodies?

Cows - meat, steak, meat loaf, hamburgers, beef – from a cow's body back part
Chicken – meat body parts, or whole chicken, wings, chest, thigh, legs–from a chicken's body
Chicken eggs – from a chicken's female body, that's their baby chicken in the egg
Chicken mayonnaise – it has eggs in it – egg whites - from a chicken body
Turkey –meat from a turkey, bird – wings, chest, thigh, legs, from a turkey's body
Pigs – meat of pork, bacon, ribs, pork roast, sausage, hot dog, bologna, ham - from a pig's body back part
Fish – meat of fish sticks, fish burgers, salmon, halibut, sushi- from a fish's body
Crab – meat from a crab's body
Lobster – meat from lobster tail– from a lobster's body
Crawfish– meat from a crawfish's body

Lamb – meat from a sheep's body

Bee honey –an insect, that eats the pollen, from a flower, put the pollen on its legs, and mixes pollen with saliva, for its baby

Could We Stop Using, Animal Leather Skin, and Animal Suede Skin Products? Not leather animal items.

leather skins of a cow clothes: leather hats, leather vests, leather coats, leather pants, leather skirts, leather belts, leather gloves

leather or swade skins of a cow shoes

leather skins of a cow purses, leather wallets, leather bags, leather dream catchers, wall plaques, and other leather items

leather skins of a cow sofas, chairs, rugs, trash cans, curtains, bed blankets

leather skins of a cow car seats, and leather motorcycles

feathers of birds, fur of animals, wool of sheep, imitation fur, animal fabric prints, or animal pictures for clothes or items

fur of rabbits, mink, fox, and other animals

Instead of using cow skins leather, Could we use vinyl, fabric materials, all man made, to make clothes, shoes and items?

Could you invite yourself to stop drinking and eating, the milk fluids, milk foods, and meat of animals?

Could we Stop using Kitchen Cooking Machines, on our food, and eat them new, they way they are, with out this?

Not at all, or don't use so much of: ovens, pots on stoves, microwaves, blenders, juicers, processors, mixers, toasters, toaster ovens.

It is too hot for the food, and it takes out of the food: energy, enzymes, nutrients, vitamins, fiber, protein, and color.

It's best to not cook food. Could we eat food fresh, and keep the food on the counters, instead of in cold refrigerators?

Could we keep the food at room temperature, like on a farm nature's temperature, instead of in the cold refrigerator?

What Could We Do, in Our Lives Nicer?

Could we eat garden and farm foods, be happy and at peace. And could we invest our money, in purchasing garden and farm foods, and purchase land, and plant fruit trees, nut trees, and bottle water, and sell that to the people, for food and items. That is wealth. We should grow cotton, linen, fleece, velvet, and vinyl, for clothes, shoes, and other items.

Could we use vinyl, man made materials, and synthetic materials for shoes, furniture, and cars and sell that to the people. That is wealth. That would be nice for us all, as an individual, couple, family, city, and countries. Our world would be a better place for we, and for the animals, to life, and be happy now, and in our future. We will be happy eating, garden and farm foods only. And the animals will be happy, if we don't eat them. Eat plants and food from the trees and plants only, of the land.

Learn about eating, fresh garden and farm food, as a new food person, and apply it to our lives, and do that. Could we live it? And then teach each other, to improve their life, by sharing your example, and inform others about changing eating habits, to a new way of eating new food, new from the garden, of the earth's land, farms, fields of fruit trees, fresh and drink water from the kitchen sink, or bottled. And dress ourselves with earth materials, of clothes and shoes, of cotton, linen, fleece, velvet fabric, and vinyl materials. Use vinyl or fabric cars, trucks, and furniture of sofas and chairs. All for a better way of life. And, save the animals of stress, worry, pain, and death. All restaurants, should stop selling animal meat and dairy, and sell only vegetarian and vegan new foods.

The nicest way to eat, drink, and life, is to eat only plant foods. Could we eat new? New fruits, new vegetables, drink pure water from the kitchen sinks filtered on the counter, or bottled. It is pure there and not cold or hot. The water is just right from the sink or bottled, at nature's temperature, of how water is to be drank, not too cold and not too hot. And some bottled water has too much writing on the bottle, and has too many pictures on the bottles. We should drink from glasses that have no writing on the glass, or pictures to get pure drinking water. Pour the bottled water into a glass and drink it clear, with out words on the glass.

This is the nicest information, we could receive for ourselves, and to teach and inform someone else, of how to eat plant and tree foods. How to eat garden foods. How to eat farm foods. How to eat orchard foods. And how to eat field foods. All from the food stores, of the fruit, vegetable, foods that is displayed there, with all the beautiful colors, and fresh enzymes, vitamins, protein, calcium, minerals, fiber, and water, in the foods for our bodies.

The most important thing that we can do, is drink water, and eat plant and tree foods from the earth, land, gardens, farms, fields, orchards, for our body and life. We eat three times a day, and we should only eat only plant and tree food for our body. We should not eat animals. We are not meant to eat animal's bodies, or drink animals milk fluids.

Could we realize this, and change our minds, change our purchasing from animals meat and animals, milk to new foods of the gardens and farms, and change our eating habits, to eat only from plants and trees, that have fruits and vegetables?

Could we could learn how to plant a fruit tree, then we can have fruit every year, as long as the tree can give its fruit, for us, to eat each year. If we eat an animal, then we have no food, after that, or the next year, because there are no seeds in animals, to plant and grow. And there are seeds in plant and tree foods, for us to eat, plant, water, and grow to eat for life.

We should stop stealing the animals, stop owning the animals, stop death the animals, stop cutting the animals up, stop taking the animal's milk fluids from them, and stop taking the flesh meat from the animal's bodies. We should stop manufacturing the animal's bodies, and milk fluids, into food and drinks, for meat and milk drinks and food items. We should stop taking the animals skins from their body, and making cow leather skin items? Could we stop selling the animals for food, clothes, pants, skirts, shirts, shoes, belts, coats, vests, hats, gloves, furniture of sofas, chairs, and rugs, car seats, truck seats, motorcycles seats and bags, dream catchers, and other items? Could we stop hurting animals?

We must realize that the animals are not food, or items. The animals are not ours to steal, own, hurt, death, sell, eat, drink, ware, or make items out of them. It's a mistake, and we have to fix it. We get to fix it, by leaving the animals alone, and let the animals be free on the land, where they belong, not in us, not in our bodies, not in our homes, not in our refrigerators, freezers, cupboards, pantries, not on the table, not on our plates, not in our toilets, or in the sewers, and not in our mouths or stomachs.

The animals want to be left alone, in nature. The animals belong to the land. We should not touch the animals, for meat and dairy milk, leather, feathers, fur, or wool products. Animals have a right to live. We should let them be free. If you ate the animal's meat items foods, wore them, or sat on them, then you ate their worry, sadness, depression, pain, death, of their bodies meat and fluids milk. And that causes us, to have those same problems, that the animals had. If the animal is sad and has a virus, that was eaten, by us, then if we ate that animal that was sad and had a virus, then we will be sad and have a virus. So if we eat foods that are free, still, quiet and kind, we will be free, still, quiet, and kind in our lives.

How to change our body, from all animal meat, and milk body, to a plant and tree, new foods of: fruits, vegetables, and water body.

If we have eaten meat, milk drinks, and milk foods, that is all from animals, mostly cows. Could we stop doing that? Could we change our body from eating animal, meat and milk, to eating from trees and plants, from the land and earth? Could we stop eating and drinking animal's bodies and milks, from the animals, and start eating plants of fruits and vegetables, and drinking new water? Animal meat and milk has animal blood in that. Garden and farm food has water in that, of the land and earth.

If you want to feel better, all you have to do is stop eating all animal meat, animal cow milk, and animal cow dairy milk drinks and milk foods. And you will lose that weight of the animals, in your body, the animals will leave away. The extra weight that you have, is mostly the animals bodies, that you ate, and are having a difficult time letting leave of the animals, of the animal's bodies, and the animal's fluids, from your body. We have to say bye, and let the animals leave. We get to let the animals leave from we, from our body, back to the land where they are from. The animals are not from we. The animals are from the land. Could we stop eating animal's meat bodies, and stop drinking animals milk fluids, and eating milk foods? That would be nice.

If we stop eating cooked foods, that may cause us to gain weight and feel sick. And if you do eat cooked foods, eat mostly cooked foods, with no animal meat, or dairy milk, or milk foods of milk, cheese, whey, sour cream, and others. We must remember that animal's meat, or dairy milk foods, are not food. Meat and dairy milk is animals. So if we stop eating animals, we will lose all the weight that we want to, and be average again. And could you keep a food journal, of your progress, with the weight loss, and new food eating habits, of eating from the garden and farm new foods, and not eating animal foods and less cooked foods. You will notice the difference. It will happen for you.

You will lose weight fast, of the animal's bodies and fluids, that you ate, and drank, and leave the animals away from you, forever, never to be eaten by you. Even if you are average weight, you still need to change your body from animal's body to fruit, vegetable and water body. Could you eat fruit and vegetables with water to drink?

The path to feeling better, is to simply stop eating animal items, and eat less cooked foods, and eat more new foods of fruit, vegetables, all new, and water from the sink filtered or bottled water poured into a glass to not drink words on the bottle. It is very easy to do.

Could we stop eating one animal? Practice not eating it. If it is pig, then stop eating all pig meats. And work on stop eating the pig for two days, for a week, for a month, and for a year. Then pick the next animal to stop eating like fish. And work on stopping eating fish for the next month. And then pick another animal to stop eating, like cow meat, and dairy milk items, and work on not eating cow for two days, a week, a month, and then a year. While your not eating animals, eat the fruits and vegetables, and water.

Could we work on stop eating the animals, until we have accomplished stopped eating all animals, for a few hours, days, weeks, months, and years? And then we will have done it, and we will have lost all of the weight that we wanted to just by stopping eating animals. Could we think that it is done already, and it will be finished. This is very easy to do, stop eating animals meats, and milk dairy drinks, and milk foods like butter, cheese, sour cream, cottage cheese, ranch, whey, chocolate, and candy, because there is so much more other foods to eat, that are healthier, and lighter, than the heavy meat and dairy milk foods.

We will feel better and lose weight effortlessly without exercise. Walking is nice a few times a week around the block. No strenuous exercise is necessary. And drink a lot of water, at least 1 cup of water at each meal. Drink what you could, even if it is just sips. You should lose several pounds a week, without eating animals, and be the weight you want to be soon.

If we stop eating cooked food, the sickness, weight, sadness will leave away. Could we stop eating breads so much, and eat new wheat or almonds. Instead of using butter, use olive oil, or dairy free butter. Instead of drinking cow milk, use soy milk, or almond nut milk. To stop eating and drinking, all animal meat and dairy milks, you will lose all the unwanted weight, that you have on your body, and it will leave away, because it is animals and not you. This is better for we in our life, in our homes, and it the citys.

Could you stop using your old glass, plates, forks, knives, and spoons that you ate animals on? Could you buy a new glass, plate, fork, knife, and spoon for your fresh garden and farm foods? Could do this in your new life, of plant based eating daily, every day? Thank you.

Cooked Foods for Vegetarians and Vegans, with no animal products in the food. Could you read the ingredients, to see if there is no milk, milk foods, or meat in them?

Oatmeal – plain or with olive oil, brown sugar, or maple syrup or soy milk, add raisons

Grits – with dairy free butter, or coconut oil

Hash browns

Potatoe Chips – plain, with no cheese, or sour cream

Humus and bread or crackers – plain, with no cheese, sour cream, or milk

Spaghetti and sauce - with no meat or cheese

Baked Potatoe - with olive oil, no butter or sour cream, use vegan butter

Veggie burger and fries – at the store, or a local fast food restaurant, with no mayonnaise it has eggs

Pizza - with vegan dairy free cheese, extra sauce, mushrooms, tomatoes, black olives

Steamed vegetables – only for about 5 minutes

Canned Fruit and canned Vegetables

Rice

Avocado Rice rolls

Falafels

Tofu

Vegetable soups – could you read the ingredients, to make sure it contains no milk or meat

Vegan chocolate chip cookies - make sure it says vegan, and contains no eggs or milk

Olives black

Halmony corn

Crackers

Bread, bagels - with dairy free butter, use olive oil, or hummus
Water and lemon
Fruit Juice
Vegetable Juice
Soy Milk plain - or Soy Milk Vanilla, Rice Milk, Coconut Milk, Almond Milk, Cashew Milk, or Oat Milk
Granola cereal with the soy milk - instead of cow milk
Granola bars -peanut butter bars, with no chocolate, or milk
Peanut butter and jelly sandwiches
Almond butter and jelly sandwiches
Red beans and rice - and barbeque sauce
Veggie burritos - with rice, beans, tomatoes, avocado, and sauce, no meat, cheese, or sour cream
Fruit pies - that contain no eggs in the crust
Cookies - that contain no milk, or eggs, vegan cookies
Grilled cheese sandwich – vegan dairy free cheese and vegan dairy free butter
Chips and salsa, chips without sour cream or cheese

After you eat vegetarian, or vegan of these foods cooked. For breakfast eat fruit, for lunch eat vegetables, and dinner cooked foods.
Then be a new food person and only eat fruits and vegetables no seeds, with water, nothing cooked.

Kitchen Cooking Equipment Machines, I don't use so much.

microwaves, blenders, juicers, processors, spiral slicer, mixers, toasters, bbq, ovens, toaster oven, stoves, pots, refrigerators, freezers.

Microwaves – Puts electricity, sound, and light into the food of vegetables, and already cooked foods, too hot for the food.

Blenders – Cuts up the solid food of fruits, vegetables, and nuts, and blends food into liquid, with water. Eat solid foods.

Juicers - Juices the solid food up and blends to liquid. Divides solid fruits and vegetables into liquid and pulp.

You don't eat the pulp. Eat solid foods and drink water.

Food Processors – They cut up the solid food into smaller pieces, easier to eat. Eat solid foods.

Spiral Slicer – Cuts the vegetables into a long noodle shape, easier to eat. Eat solid foods.

Electric Mixers – We are not supposed to make our food and cook it, the garden and farm already made foods new of fruits and vegetables.

Toasters or Toaster Ovens – Too hot for our food, electricity gets into the bread and bagels.

Barbeques – Too hot for our food.

Ovens – Too hot for our food. Electricity gets into food.

Stoves Pots – Too hot, electricity gets into the food. Use for only 5 minutes to lightly steam vegetables. Eat new foods instead.

Refrigerator and Freezer– Could you not use the refrigerator, and put your food on the counter, to keep the food at Nature's

temperature, like the food was on the gardens and farms, for several months, on the land plant or on a tree. The refrigerator is dark all day and all night, the foods need natural sunlight in our kitchen, so keep them on the counter. The refrigerator is too cold and has electricity and sound, that is put into the foods, it takes out the natural sunlight they absorbed, for all that time on the land. And try to not freeze your foods. Keep them new on the counter. Could you put a white shelf where the refrigerator was for your food, and water bottles and water containers?

Recipe Books – That food is mostly cooked, baked, blended, juiced, processed, animal items, or cut up, not solid.

All of those kitchen cooking machines, have electricity to run them. The electricity gets into the foods, and causes problems. Too cold causes colds or the flu. Too hot causes fevers. Electricity on our food causes us problems when we eat them, sicknesses. Try to eat the foods without the use of machines. Don't change foods, eat them the way they are: solid, still, quiet, and free.

Gardens and Farms, Plants and Trees Foods, of the Land and Earth –

Could you eat fresh foods of fruits and vegetables, uncooked, not spin, made into liquid, without machines? It's the nice to eat the food in solid form, as it was made on the farms and gardens, still and quiet.

Our food is already made in the garden and farms, new, not cooked, or all cut up by equipment machines, or cut up by someone else. Don't purchase already cut up food, by the store that someone else cut up. Purchase the food solid, and peel it yourself, or cut it yourself, if you have to. Buy more food that you can peel, or eat, and cut yourself. It is better like that.

The food is already cooked, buy the sun, for months. We don't have to cook it again, after that. It is already cooked, for us, the how it is: fruits and vegetables, with water.

Could you eat your garden and farm foods, without the use of kitchen equipment machines, as much as possible?

1. Some fruits and vegetables you can eat
2. Some fruits and vegetables you peel
3. Some fruits and vegetables require cutting them, with a knife, and that is the most we should use on our foods.

Foods and Beverages, that I don't eat, as a Fresh Food Person

cooked foods – causes sicknesses, depression, sad, tired, overweight, eat new foods

salt and pepper or spices, they are cooked, and dried, not new

bread - its cooked in an oven, and it's too hot

croissants – it has eggs and milk in that

sugar - it's a man made product, not natural

candy – too much sugar and chocolate with cow milk in it

hamburgers – it is cow meat, eat a veggie burger

vinegar - it is fermented, old, preserved

ranch– they have vinegar, or milk in it, just eat the spinach or lettuce plain

chocolate - it has cow milk in it

doughnuts - it has milk and eggs

cookies - they have chocolate, egg, milk, and sugar

soda drinks – they have carbonation, and are man made products, drink water

energy drinks - they have carbonation, and man made products, drink water

sushi – it is fish or crab

pies of fruit– the ingredients say eggs, it must be in the crust

pizza – it has cheese - from a cow, and meat from a cow or pig

gum- we don't need to do that, just get something to eat instead

almond butter – it is cooked nuts

peanut butter – it is cooked nuts

citric acid – it is in pickles, and olives, and some orange juice, it ferments the food

honey – from the bees, they make it for their family, not for we

eggs – from chickens birds

potato chips – not with sour cream, or cheese from cows

food in jars – it is preserved, instead of new

food in boxes – it is dried, instead of new

soup – someone else cut up the vegetables, not whole foods, find vegan soups, that contain no milk or meat

food in cans – it is cut up, and in the dark can, for who knows how long, and preserved

animal meat or dairy products – its dead animals, causes sickness, hair loss, weight gain, pain, aches, and others

alcohol, wine, or wine coolers, champagne - it is fermented grapes, it is a liquid drug, eat grapes and drink water

beer – it is fermented barley wheat grain, it is a liquid drug, eat wheat new

coffee - it has caffeine-a drug, the bean is cooked, crushed up, and blended, cooked, too hot, drink water

caffeine tea- it has caffeine, -a drug, too hot, drink water

cigarettes – dried leaves, artificial smoke air, it is a drug, eat some spinach

medications – it is man made artificial, and it is a drug, causes hair loss, restless leg syndrome, only take aspirin or tums

vitamins – it is man made, eat the garden new food, they have all the vitamins and minerals

If you want to be a plant and tree, new food person, eat and drink new foods only of: fruits and vegetables, and water.

Could We Stop Wearing, Dead Animal Leather Skin Products, of Clothes, Shoes, or Items?

Not leather, suede, fur, imitation fur, feathers, or wool products, that were taken from animal's skin bodies,

cut or plucked off of them. It is their body, not ours. That hurts the animals. That's sad.

leather shoes –it is cow skin, could we wear fabric, vinyl, and all man made materials for shoes leather coats – it is cow skin

leather vests – it is cow skin

leather pants, skirts – it is cow skin

leather or swede tool belt or work belts - it is cow skins, use vinyl or fabric

leather hats – it is cow skin

leather wallets – it is cow skin, use fabric wallets, vinyl wallets, or an envelope

leather purses or bags – it is cow skin, use fabric or vinyl materials

leather gloves – it is cow skin

leather car seats or truck seats, and motorcycle seats and bags – it is cow skins, taken off of the cow's body, use fabric or vinyl

leather furniture of sofas, chairs, rugs, trash cans, curtains, bed blankets – it is cow skins, use fabric materials

animal wall mounts, stuffed animals, animal toys – don't use, throw away

suede shoes – its leather, cow skin, taken off of the animal's body, use fabric or vinyl

fur coats – its animals skin and fur, taken off of the animal's body

fur hats – it is animal skin and fur

imitation fake fur coats - it looks like animals fur, yet it is man made materials

imitation fake fur blankets and pillows - it looks like animals fur, yet it is man made materials

feather pillows – its bird's wings, pulled out of the bird

feather comforter – its bird's wings arms

feathers in the hats – its bird's wings arms

feather coats – it is birds wings, plucked off the bird

feather dream catchers – feathers from birds

rabbit fur coats – it is rabbit's skins and fur, cut off of the animal's body

rabbit foots - key chains, it's animals body parts

mink fur coats – it is animal's skin and fur, cut off of the animal's body

wool – it is sheep fur, cut off of the sheep's body

Animals fabric material prints and fabric pictures of animals- don't use

----

All of those animals have suffered, that were made into food, clothing, shoes, car seats, or furniture of sofas, chairs, rugs,

and accessories. It is wrong and sad. Could we stop doing that and use earth items? That is nicer.

Could we use cotton, linen, fleece, velvet, and vinyl fabrics – natural from the land earth grown on farms?

Could we read the labels, to purchase fabric shoes, vinyl shoes, and all man made materials, stated on the shoe?

Could we ask a sales person, to show you where the fabric shoes and all vinyl shoes are, in the store?

Only solid colors on clothes, shoes, food, drinks, or items – not numbers, faces of people, children's pictures, animals, buildings, nature scenes, logos, names of people, or name brands on the outside of the clothes, rips, holes, or other problems on the clothes or items.

Instead of investing our money in dead animal items, could we invest our money, into life garden and farm, earth materials and garden foods of seeds, fruit trees, nut trees, vegetarian food, vegan foods, new foods, cotton, linen, fleece, velvet, and vinyl, and other fabric of materials, that are earth friendly, made from the land of farms, instead of using animal's body skins called leather, feathers, fur, or wool?

We already have skin, we don't need to wear the skins of cows, or other animals on our body. Thank You.

New Garden and Farm Foods, and Pure Water

New garden and farm foods cause us to have a healthy life, alive, sense better, happy, new, ideas, free, decisions, improvement, positive attitudes, peace, achieve ideas, spiritual, kind, awake, wake up, awareness, meditate, and others ideas. Our belief, dreams, ideas, life, and work should all be in Nature, and in the Garden, and Farm Foods of Fruit and Vegetables, and Water of the land and of the Earth's gardens, farms, fields, orchards, trees and plants, and also use vinyl, cotton, fleece, velvet, and linen clothes, shoes and items. Home, Family, Work, taking a Walk, Eating and Drinking Healthy, and Rest is what we could think about, do, and be like for all of our life.

From the start of Time, to eat only garden and farm food, is the best law of old time. Yet, something happened wrong and sad, and some of them they stopped eating only garden and farm foods, and they started eating cooked foods, and animal foods, and wearing animal clothes, and making animal furniture, cars, and trucks, and items. We as a people, as a world, as a country, as a city, as a home, as an individual, must get back to only eating garden foods and stop eating and drinking animal meat and dairy items. We must stop wearing animal skins, and making items with their skins like shoes, chairs, sofas, car seats, motorcycles, bags, purses, earrings, wallets, belts, gloves, and hats and other items.

Food stores are now about 70% animal products and 30% Garden and Farm food.

We need our Food Stores to be 100% Garden and Farm foods.

No animals in the building stores, the animals belong on the land. Not in our mouths, stomachs, bodies, toilets, or homes.

Animal food products have blood in it. We don't want to eat, or drink, animal milk drinks with blood, from them being cut up. Blood meat and blood milk, is in animal meats and dairy milk and meat. All sicknesses, viruses, and diseases, are from eating animal items, and too much cooked foods. We should eat more new fruits and vegetables, in our life, on earth now today and forever.

Garden food has water in it, minerals, vitamins, enzymes, fiber, protein, calcium, and life energy.

Animal items of milk, dairy items, and animal meat, has blood in it, stress and worry of the animal.

Cooked foods are devitalized and dehydrated of water, and causes the food color to be dull, and causes the life to leave out of the food. Eating cooked foods is like eating cut up pieces of paper, it really doesn't do anything for us except fill us up, hurt us, and makes us sick, and hungry. Eating cooked foods causes us to keep eating, because we aren't eating new foods, and the cooked foods keep us wanting to eat more and more. Cooked foods don't have oxygen in them, and we need oxygen to life ourselves. So, eat foods that have oxygen in them like fruits, vegetables, nuts, grains, and water.

Could we eat the fruit and vegetables, in solid form? Like eating a whole apple, or a whole tomato. Yet, you cannot eat a whole cow, or you cannot eat a whole pig, and you cannot eat a whole chicken, because it is too big. We are not suppose to eat animals, because they have faces, arms, legs, tail, fur, feathers, or wool. Could we stop eating meat with a face on it? Don't eat anything with a face on it, or eyes on it. Don't eat anything that has arms and legs on it, of the animals.

Could we eat only the garden and farm foods that have leaves, a stem, leaves, and seeds in them. That is safe. Take the seeds out, and plant the seeds in the ground in your back yard at home. That will be a nice experience to grow your own food and eat that, fun.

One person can eat an apple, or a tomato individually, and be healthy and happy. Yet, many people have eaten from a cow and shared it. You can't eat a whole cow as one person, it is too much and shouldn't be done anyway. Maybe 50 people ate off of one cow and caught a virus, from eating that cow, and was sick. Because eating from and animal makes us we with sickness.

If you want to be a real garden and farm New Food Person, then purchase and eat only new food to eat. And shop at the stores, at the local new food stores, where they only sell garden and farm foods, and they do not sell dead animal meats, and live animal dairy milk. The food is mostly out for you to shop and not refrigerated. This is nice for the food, and for us to eat. Could you experiment, and purchase only garden and farm foods, for one week, and eat garden and farm foods for a week, and see how it sense for you? That would be nice. And you may notice an improvement in yourself, and in your life in what you do, and feeling better. Save the animals, and save the plant, and save the world, and save the people from viruses, by eating plants and trees food of fruits and vegetables, and life healthy. Thank You

Cooked Foods, Animal Meat, and Animal Dairy Milk Drinks and Milk Foods

Cooked foods, meat and dairy milk cause us to feel sick, tired, stomach hurts, body hurts, head aches, problems, sad, hallucinations, doubt, wrong thinking, wrong actions, false traditions, depression, over sleep, irritated, upset, dizzy, cancer, angry, hair loss, acne, colds, flu, rashes, throw up, heart attacks, viruses, and other problems of health concerns. All of our problems are due to eating food the wrong and sad path, such as eating dead animal's meat, drinking alive animal's milk, eating too much cooked foods, juiced, blended, spiral sliced, canned, boxed, microwaved, oven, toaster ovens, or pots on the stove foods. So, could we eat fresh fruits and vegetables with water only every day of our lifes on earth either 100%, or 80% fruits and vegetables new not cooked, and cooked foods about 20%. This will be best for us as a world of people. We should try to stay away from eating 3 cooked meals a day, to only 1 cooked meal a day, and the other 2 meals new fruits and vegetables all fresh. Remember that cooked foods don't have oxygen in them. And you would be depriving your body of oxygen from the fruits and vegetables and nuts with water. Try that.

How to get started, and what to do?

Try for one day, to stop eating cooked foods, and animal meats, and animal milk products, and only eat new garden and farm foods of fruits and new vegetables, and water only. See how you feel about it. Test it out and do that. You might like it better eating new, instead of eating cooked and animal's foods. Then you can be another day, and a week, a month and a year. This is called a new food person.

We must leave and stop, the dead animal body flesh meat eating, and animal cow milk fluids drinking old world behind, and start a new world of eating only garden and farm foods, and drinking only water, today, now, and forever . This is best for us we, and for the world.

If you have any dead animals, meat or milk products, could we throw it away, and clean out the refrigerator and freezer?

Could we throw away:
animal meat foods
animal dairy milk drinks
animal boxed foods
animal canned foods
animal dried foods
animal food in jars
animal frozen foods

animal microwave foods

plates, bowls, glasses, and utensils of forks, knifes, spoons, that you ate and drank, animal milk, and meat foods, out of containers,

that stored or used animal meat, and dairy milk drinks and milk foods.

trash cans, that had dead animal meat or dairy products in it, and purchase a new trash can

Could you purchase a new refrigerator, with no dead animal products in that, refrigerator on top and freezer on the bottom.

Or throw your refrigerator away and use only the counters to put your foods, like they grew on the farm.

Could you buy all new kitchen towels, plates, bowls, glasses, utensils of forks, knifes, spoons, garbage can, table and chairs that are

only for new garden foods, no animal food on that.

If you have animal leather, fur, feathers, wool: clothes, shoes, items, could you throw them away?

leather clothes, pants, skirts, shirts, vests, coats, gloves, jewelry, and shoes. Could you get new clothes, and new shoes fabric?

leather, sofas and chairs, and buy new furniture and car truck, motorcycle seats, of vinyl or fabric, sofas and chairs.

Could you buy new clothes that are fabric, and shoes that are fabric, or vinyl, all man made materials and synthetic?

If you can afford it, buy a new home, where only fresh garden foods will be, and no dead animals in the house.

Could you buy all new white towels, rugs, and furniture that is new, and not used from touching the animals.

You will have a new life, eating garden, and farm food. And you will notice the difference, is nice and free.

If you have a leather car, could you take it to the car yard, and sell it for a few hundred dollars, and purchase a new

car with fabric, or vinyl seats, instead if you can afford, to do that. Or trade your leather car in for a fabric car. You will feel better about it.

Don't pass on your animal clothes, or animal items to someone else, for money, throw it away, and start new.

If you have a leather sofa or chairs, have it picked up by the city trash, and could you buy a fabric sofa and chair new?

Could we eat new foods, instead of dried fruit, and dried vegetables, or cooked fruit, and cooked vegetables.

A New Life

Could we plant a garden or farm, in the back yard of fruit and vegetables? Purchase the seeds and plant them, or purchase the plants at the plant stores, and plant them, water them, and pick them new to eat. Grapefruit, apples, pears, oranges, cantaloupe, tomatoes, spinach, avocados, potatoes. And other foods. All you have to do is water them after you plant them, and pick the food. It is new and healthy. It is nice to do, and it's natural to the earth and land.

Could you eat healthy of new foods, sit and think, take a walk in nature, plant a garden, work, clean, talk, and rest? That is all. Keep that all garden and farm foods, new from the land to eat, and plant clothes to wear.

This is all a new way of life, and will bring you closer, to how you may want to be, and life.

Try this and see how it is for you, I am sure you will like it better.

In this way we can improve our selves, our city, our world and our earth, on our planet and in our universe.

We can give back animals their rights, by not eating them, and letting them be free on the land, not in our bodies, and not in our mouths.

And we can be more of the nicest, and free, by eating only new garden and farm foods.

What you can do, is stop eating at least one animal body meat, or dairy milk fluid drinks, and see how that is for you.

Then work on the next animal item, until you eventually stop eating, all animal items, of meat and dairy milk and milk foods.

Or, you can just stop eating all animal items at once, and become a new food person, eating garden and farm food.

Could we work on this for a day, of first eating only garden and farm foods and water? Then work on it for another day, and then a week, month, and a year, and then for the rest of our life. And then continuing on into the next life, when we die, and travel to the spirit world of people in heaven, and eat of fruits and vegetables there. The animals will be happy for us doing this, and we will be happy for doing this, forever of eating new foods only.

Could we look at the new food in the stores, it is all new, not cooked, it has many colors. If you have seen a rainbow, it has many colors, and so does our food. We should eat all of the different fruits and vegetables, of all of various size, shape, and color.

We have a rainbow of foods. We have red apples, orange oranges, yellow squash, green spinach, blue berries, purple cabbage, white banana, and black blackberries. All colors of the rainbow.

It takes practice eating new food every day, and for the rest of your life, in a world that sells animal products. We have to stay in the food stores, to purchase our food, and keep new foods in our homes, restaurants, businesses, fuel stations, convient stores, fruit stands, and other places.

Could we do a test, and experiment, to eat only new and garden foods, not cooked, roasted, salted, blended, juiced, mixed, baked in ovens, or on stoves in pots, and eat the food of fruit and vegetables new, for one day. And see how you sense for the day, and then try for another day. And then a week and month, and then a year without. You will notice a difference in your life doing this.

It is important to stop eating all animal meat: of cows, chickens, pigs, fish, turkey, bee, shrimp, crawfish, crab, lobster, deer, lamb and other animals.

It is important to stop drinking milk of cows: 1%, 2%, Whole Milk, and Half and Half milk.

It is important to stop eating milk dairy products, from cows of: cheese, yogurt, ice cream, sour cream, cottage cheese, whey, ranch, chocolate, and candy.

It is important to stop eating eggs and mayonnaise from chickens birds.

It is important to stop wearing cow skin leather: of pants, shirts, shirts, vests, coats, belts, wallets, purses, gloves, and hats.

It is important to stop making and sitting on leather skin sofas and chairs or office chairs, and not walking on animal fur rugs.

It is important to stop making and driving in cow animal skin leather cars, trucks, motorcycle, or boat seats.

Did you know about an Apple to Eat?

Do you know the process that it takes, for you to have an Apple to eat?
All you have to do is, pick from the tree, and eat the apple.
That is if you have an apple tree.

If you don't have an apple tree, then you may have to do the following:

Take the seeds from an apple,
plant the seeds in the ground,
water the seeds and trees,
wait for the tree to grow fruits, apples,
pick an apple on the farm tree,
put the apple in a basket,
drive the apples in a basket to the store,
put the apples on the self to sell,
pick out an apple that you want to eat,
put the apple in a bag,
put the apple in a basket,
purchase the apple at the food store,
put the apple in your car,
take the apple home with you,
wash the apple off,
dry the apple off with a napkin or paper towel,
and eat the apple.
Feel happy and nice.
Have seeds to grow another apple tree for food.

This is very right and nice to do, if you are hungry for an apple, and safe to eat.
No animals were hurt in the process of this.
Nature is our inspiration.
This is natural.
This is the way it should be.
This is how all of our food should be.
This is the healthy way.
This is divine.
This is a high form of living.
This is a high form of eating.
This is a new food person.
This is the new way.

Did you know about, animal cow milk, and animal cow meat, to Not drink, or eat?

Hunted for a cow,

stole a cow,

captured a cow, from its land,

took the cow, to your land,

made the cow, get into a work truck,

drove the cow, to a business of animals building,

took the cow, out of the work truck,

took the cow, into the building,

put a milking machine, on the cow, to get the milk -white blood fluid milk dairy, out of the cow, for cow milk drinks and milk foods,

the cow died in the building,

cut all the cow, up for meat food

cut the cow sides and back, up for animal skins leather clothes, shoes, furniture, and automobiles, and other items,

sent the meat food of the cow, to the manufactures, to make the meat food, cut up into cans, boxes, and saran rap,

sold the cow meat food, to the people, in the food stores, and restaurants, and stores,

sold the cow skins leather to clothing stores, shoes stores, and car stores, for leather items,

purchased and took home, the cow meat food,

cooked, the cow meat food,

ate, the cow, body meat food,

drank, the cow, milk liquid,

felt sick, pain, throw up, overweight, cancer, virus, and flu, blind, other problems.

This is wrong and sad.

This is the old way, of a false tradition, that must be stopped. Stopped with you first, then tell others.

Could you not drink cow's milk?

Could you not eat cow's meat?

Could you not wear cow's skin leather or swede?

Be nice to the cows, take care of them.

It's much easier to eat an apple, and nicer.

To:
The Businesses of Hunters of Land, Ocean, and Air Animals
The Businesses of Animals Manufactures of Milk
The Businesses Animals Manufactures of Meat
The Businesses of Food Stores of Animals Milk and Animal Meat
The Business of Stores that sell animal clothes and shoes, cars and trucks, wallets and purses, and other items

Could you stop hunting animals, and plant seeds, on farms and gardens, and harvest fresh food to sell instead?

Could you stop selling animals, to people, to death, hurt, cut up, to sell for food, and drinks?

Could you stop selling dead animal's meat flesh, and alive animal's milk fluids, to eat and drink, to people? Could you close, your business of animals, and manufacturing businesses of animal's bodies meat and animals milk fluids,

for one day, during the week, to see how it is, without that process, and then for a week, and for a month, and year, and permanently? Thanks

Could you let the cows and animals, be free in nature, and stop owning them, and death them, and selling them for food

and drinks? Instead of using the animal buildings, could you close them, and take them down to the ground and throw away, to stop viruses?

Could you buy new land, build a new metal building, buy all new foods, of the farm and gardens of new fruit and new vegetables, and water, and sell that to the people in a food store?

Could you only sell garden farm foods, and not sell any dead animal meat, and live animal dairy milk, and dead animal milk foods?

Could you buy land, and plant, fruit trees, nut trees, and vegetables, for the food store?

We need more food stores, with garden and farm foods, and no animal foods or animal drinks.

Could you prepare vinyl, and synthetic materials, and fabrics, for shoes, car seats, and furniture of sofas, chairs and rugs in a furniture store?

What to do as a city, concerning food, and the animals?

Could we stop purchasing, all dead animal meats, and animal cow, dairy milk drinks, and milk foods?

Could we have food stores, that sell only life garden and farm foods, and not sell dead animal items?

Could we shop at local food stores, who sell mostly fruits and vegetables, and water?

We could stop purchasing meats, on holidays, and eat only garden and farm foods? It's a false tradition to eat dead animal foods.

If we could get the hunters of birds, hunters of land animals, and hunters of ocean animals, to stop hunting and fishing, and bringing that dead animal meat, filled with blood, to eat, our lives would be better, and more free as a country. We don't want to eat that ever. It is wrong and sad. And we could get those people, new work, with gardens foods, to help improve our countries and city, and feed us better, from the gardens and farms of fruits and vegetables, and water.

We could get the businesses of hunters, business of animals, and manufactures of animal bodies meats, and dairy cow milk fluids, to stop hunting, and fishing, the animals, and death them, and to close their places, and take the buildings down to the ground and throw away that, and let the animals be free. How can we help the animals? How can we help those people, who had to do that to the animals? How can we help ourselves, who had to eat the animals, and drink the animals?

Eating healthy, takes practice, in a world that mostly eats, dead animals meat bodies, and drinks animals milk fluids, and eats milk dairy drinks, of cheese and butter, and other dairy products, for breakfast, lunch, dinner, and snacks. Animal meat and milk, is in all kinds of foods, and must not be eaten, because it is animals, and meat and milk belongs to them. It is not ours to eat.

What about the animal's new life? How are the animals suppose to get their body back, after 50 people ate from one cow? The cow's body, if eaten by about 50 people, how it that cow, suppose to get its body back? And 30 people ate one pig meat. How is the pig receive its body back? And it doesn't want it's body back that way, all cut up, and in someone's body after eaten or drank. So let's stop eating animals, and drinking animals, and let the animals, have their body back. The animals have to wait for us to have the animals bodies leave our bodies and to give the animals bodies back to them. Sad.

And the animals don't want to get flushed down the toilet, even though the animals have to leave our body. So it is nicest that we don't eat animals, and we won't have to flush animals in the toilet, away from us. That is a problem. Who is going to be at the sewer department, to wash off the animals, that was flushed there? The animals live in the sewer for the rest of their dead lives, because of us eating them. So it is best to not eat the animals, in the first place, and only eat garden farm foods, of fruits, vegetables, and nuts. We must think of the animals and what they might have to do, before we consider eating them, and we shouldn't eat them, or flush them.

"Thank you", say the animals, for eating fruits and vegetables, and fresh water, and not eating the animals.

On the computer internet search, could you type in slaughter house videos of: cows, chickens, pigs and sheep, to see what happened to them? It is so sad what they did to them, let's stop that, and start a new life.

Could we watch videos of picking fruits and vegetables on the computer?

Could we plant fruit trees, nut trees, and vegetable plants, on the land there, out in the field, and build a new metal building, and harvest and pick the fruit, to be sold to the local food stores. This is a new idea for them, to do this for our countries, and world, of only new foods to eat.

If the hunters, fishers, slaughter houses and manufactures of animals are producing 70% of the world's food,

and farmers are producing 30% of the world's food. We need to change something.

Farmers should be producing 100% of our new foods. And could the business of animal's people, be farmers instead?

We need to stop the dead foods of animal products, and help them all change, and learn how to grow vegetation living new food, for us 100%.

Could you look around in the food stores, and see all of the new food, and stay in the new food area mostly. We don't need canned, boxed, and jars of animal foods. We need only the new fruit and vegetables, nuts, sprouts, wheat, and water. All the garden foods look like a rainbow of colors that we could eat daily.

We want to only eat garden and farm foods, from plants and trees.

We don't want to eat animal's meat bodies, or drink animal's milk fluids drinks, or milk foods.

All sicknesses, are caused from eating too much cooked foods, and animal meats, and animal milk dairy products: cancer, acne, headaches, viruses, stomach aches, overweight, vision loss, hair loss, birth defects, rashes, and other problems.

It is sad that garden and farm foods, and animal meat and milk drinks, have been mixed together in our bodies. Yet garden and farm food has to be there, to help us fix the problem, with the solution to change our body from animal's bodies and fluids, to garden and farm foods, of fruits and vegetables, and water body.

Eating vegetarian, vegan and especially new foods, will help you to wake up. You will have several awakenings, and realized some important issues in your life, and that will be amazing. You may find yourself thinking, I have woke up, and realized that I was sleeping, and now I am awake. The cooked foods and animals meats and milks caused me to be sleeping with my eyes open. Several awakenings may occur for you eating all new foods of new fruits and new vegetables, and water. You may find that you sensed that you have woke up, with a realization, because the garden and farm foods from plants and trees, helps us to wake up. Eating foods the right way, will cause us to have awakenings in our life, more frequently. We as the world of people need to wake up from the walking sleep that were in due to eating dead animals and drinking alive animals milks, and milks foods. And we wake up with fruits and vegetables with water.

Could we eat all of the foods in the area at the food store, and our life will get better, we will feel better, look better, and life better. This is all a new way of life, and garden and farm foods new, will bring you closer to how you may want to be, and life.

Could you do this, and see how it is for you, you may like it better?

In this way we can improve our selves, our citys, our countries, our world, our earth, our planet, and our universe.

We can give back animals their rights, by not eating them, and letting them be free on the land, not in our stomachs, or in our mouths.

And we can be more nice, and free, by eating only new garden and farm foods.

What you can do, is stop eating at least one animal body meat, or dairy milk fluid item, and see how that is for you.

Then work on the next animal item, until you eventually stop eating all animal's drinks and animal's foods.

Or, you can stop eating all animal items, and become a new food person, eating only garden and farm foods.

Eating some cooked food is fine, as long as the cooked food contains no animal meat or no animal milk liquids of cows of:

milk, cheese, sour cream, cottage cheese, whey, ranch, chocolate, candy, or other dairy milk liquids, or milk foods in it.

Eating only new foods, and drinking water only, will help to fill our body, with living foods, instead of dead foods, and help us, to take out the wrong and sad foods, from our body of meat and milk drinks.

Could we only purchase garden and farm fresh foods, and purchase vinyl products, or fabric items, for shoes, furniture, and cars?

As you make the money, for you, and your family, then you only purchase the garden and farm foods for your family to eat?

Could we build and design, more parks for individuals, and families, to walk with a walking paths, around the park, many trees,

and park benches, and places to like nature weekly.

Could we purchase land, and build one level homes for vegetarians, vegans, and for new food people only. Have no stoves in the kitchen, no ovens, and no refrigerator. Build more counter space for the foods. And not use so much kitchen machines of electricity items. And keep our foods on the counters, to keep the refrigeration's electricity out of the food? Thank You.

Healing

Eat Natural New Foods from the Earth
Drink Purified Water
Ware Cotton, Linen, Fleece, Velvet, and Vinyl Clothes and Shoes

What to Eat and Drink, as a New Food Person

Eat Fruits - New and solid foods, not from cans that are preserved, or already cut up from the store.

Eat Vegetables – New and solid foods, not cooked, steamed or canned.

Drink Water - From the kitchen sink filtered, or bottled. Try to not drink too much cold or hot water. Room temperature.

Clothing - Wear cotton, linen, velvet, fleece and vinyl clothes. Purchase only plain colors and not patterns or prints.
Could we not wear animal leather, suede, fur, feathers, wool, imitation fur, animal prints, and animal pictures.
Dress modestly. And wear only vinyl or fabric shoes.
Buy new white sheets, blanket, comforter, duvet, and white towels, or other colors plain.
Men wear black, white, blue, and beige. Women wear black, white, pink, red, burgandy, and beige.

Furniture - Purchase only what you need for your apartment, or house, only the basics, don't purchase extra items.
Kitchen table and chairs- metal frames, white laminate table top, white chairs metal.
Living room white or beige sofa, chairs- metal and wood frames and fabric or vinyl, not leather. Lamps, and tables.
Office desk, chair fabric or vinyl, lamp and computer.
Bedroom bed and plastic dresser, lamps, and side tables.
Not so much pictures, paintings, accessories.

Car and Truck - Purchase fabric or vinyl, new if you can, not leather seats.

Activity - Take walks, sit and think, talk, eat fresh food, drink fresh water, work, plant a garden, clean, and rest.

House – Interior Design

If you have the money, design and build your own home of a metal frame, on some land, near the woods, near nature.

Design the house further back in the land, away from the street.

Design the kitchen, and living room, to the front of the house. White fixtures.

One level house, not two levels, so no one above you, or below you.

Design the bedrooms, to the back of the home, by the back yard, for privacy with 2 walk in closets, for him and her.

Bathroom has 2 toilet in a separate room, 2 showers in a separate room, and two sinks in another room for him & her.

Laundry room by the kids rooms, with a folding table built in, hanger rack.

Laundry room for parents with two washers and dryers, and a folding table, and hanger rack.

Family room, have a white or beige sofa with two cushions love seat, for the couple, and individual chairs for each child's own chair.

Have each child's room with their own bathroom.

Couples room on one side of the house, and the kids rooms on the other side of the house.

Design and build metal and wood furniture and plastic dressers.

Carpet beige in the living room and bedrooms, white vinyl floors in the kitchen, and bathrooms, no tile so you don't have lines, beige paint.

White kitchen cupboards, and white laminate counters.

White bathroom sink, shower, and white vinyl floors all one, no lines on the floor or in the shower one solid shower walls, no lines.

Have an office for him and for her, two desks and two chairs.

Sitting area of chairs and table in the kitchen, you don't really need to have a dining room unless you want to.

Windows that open from the top and the bottom.

Use cement for outside the house on the walls, and cement roof, to be one walls and one roof, and paint the walls and roof white.

And plant a garden.

2 car garage.

Food for New Food People to Eat and Drink

Day 1 Breakfast
Grapefruit
Banana without the seeds, cut the seeds out

Lunch
Potato new, not cooked
Water

Snack
Pear

Dinner
Lettuce leafs
Avocado
Blackberries
Water

Day 2
Breakfast
Cantaloupe
Water

Lunch
Spinach
Tomato, take out the seeds
Almonds
Water

Dinner
Avocado
Apple
Water

Fruits, vegetables, nuts and how to eat them, from the garden and farms, of plants and trees, of the land and earth.

Eat the skin	Cut the skin off	no skins	peel skin off	Break the shell off
apple	watermelon	mushroom	grapefruit	almond
cherry	pineapple	pepper	orange	Peanut
asparagus	lime	cauliflower	banana	coconut
grape	avocado	spinach		
orange	melon	lettuce		
grapefruit	cantaloupe	carrot		
blueberry	lemon	brussel sprout		
pear		black olive		
peach		cabbage		
plum		broccoli		
zucchini		blackberry		
potato		raspberry		
blueberry				
sweet potato				
squash				
blueberry				
egg plant-black plant				

Animals skins that we should not eat

Could we not eat the skins of chickens, and not take off their feathers?
Could we not take off the skins of cows, and not use them for clothes, shoes, furniture, cars and trucks, and items?
Could we not take off the feathers of birds, and not use them for clothes and items?
Could we not take off the fur of animals, and not use them for coats and rugs?
Could we not take off wool of sheep, and not use them for clothes?

Food Questions

Day, Month, and Year _____

What is your weight? _____

Do you want to lose weight, and how much? _____

What foods to you like to eat?

_____

_____

What foods do you not like to eat?

_____

_____

What do you have that is animal leather, swade, feathers, fur, imitation fur, wool, animal prints, or animal pictures to throw away?

_____

_____

What cooked food, microwaved, canned, boxed, meat or dairy animal products, do you have in the kitchen, that you could throw away?

_____

What kitchen cooking machines equipment, do you have, that you could not use so much, or throw away?

_____

Does your car have leather seats, fabric, or vinyl? _____

If your car has leather seats, what other car could you buy fabric instead? _____

Do you have animal leather, furniture, or accessories?

_____

What furniture could you purchase, that is fabric or vinyl?

_____

What fresh garden and farm foods, do you like to eat?

_____

Do you have a business, that sells animal products, and what is it?

_____

What could you sell, instead of animal meat, and animal dairy milk products?

_____

_____

What animal meat, and animal milk dairy products, have you eaten?

_____

_____

What could you buy that is fabric material, vinyl, all man made materials, or synthetic materials?

_____

_____

Do you have a garden? Could you plant a garden? What fruit and nut trees could you plant?

_____

_____

_____

_____

Who could you teach, about eating only, new garden and farm foods?

_____

_____

_____

Who could you teach, about not wearing animal leather, not eating animal meat, not drinking animal milk, and not eating animals dairy milk foods?

_____

_____

If you have a Food Store, what food could you have in it, that are new, from the gardens and farms?

_____

_____

Could We Eat These Garden and Farm Foods New?

Fruit – new
Vegetables - new
Water – new, from the sink filtered, or bottled, or containers, pour into a glass the water so you don't have to drink words on the bottle.
Some Cooked Foods of Fruit and Vegetables - with no alive animal milk dairy, or dead animal meat in it.
All the fresh foods have vitamins, minerals, protein, calcium, fiber, light and color in them for us we.

Could we stop wearing cows, sheeps, and birds, and other animals, clothes, shoes, and items?

cow leather skins, cow suede skins, of clothes, shoes, wallets, purses, cars, furniture of sofas, chairs, rugs and items
bird feathers on clothes, earrings, hats and items
sheep wool made into clothes

Could we wear these fabric and materials?

Cotton, linen, fleece, velvet, vinyl, synthetic, all man made materials, fabric materials for clothes and shoes

Could We Stop Eating the Animals, Wearing the Animals, and Using the Animals Items?

Cows –dairy milk products
Cows- meat
Cows - leather skin: items of clothes, shoes, cars, trucks, motorcycles, sofas, chairs, rugs, trash cans, bed blankets, curtains, and other items
Chickens - meat
Chicken - eggs of babies
Birds - chickens, eagles – feathers - pillows, comforters, coats, and hats, dream catchers
Pigs - meat
Fish - meat
Turkey - meat
Bee – honey
Shrimp - meat
Crab - meat
Lobster -meat
Oyster – meat, pearls rings, necklaces, and jewelry. The pearls grew in the meat of the oyster.
Deer – venison meat, animal head wall mounts placks
Goat - milk

Could we stop making cooked foods, with animal's foods, of meat or milk in them?
Could we stop making, any Animal head plaques, on wall mounted frames, as trophies, and throw them all away?

Could we Start doing this?

Could we keep the fruit and vegetables and water, on the counter, at room temperature, like on the farms and gardens nature's temperature,
outside in the field, instead of in the cold refrigerators, in the dark all day, with the hot electricity from the outlet,
that changes our food, from outside temperature to cold temperature or freezing.
That is sad for the food. The food is nicest on the counters at outside temperature to keep the refrigeration hot and cold, light,
and sound out of our body if eaten from the refrigerators.
Could we eat or food from the counters, instead of in the refrigerators?
Could we purchase from stores that don't refrigerate our food, and keep them on the counters out of the refrigerators?
Could we eat fruit and vegetables, and water all new. Not cooked, canned, steamed, or dried?
Could we buy all vinyl shoes, or fabric shoes, no leather or suede in the stores?
Could we buy new items of clothes of cotton, linen, fleece, velvet, of shirts and pants, and fleece coats?
Could we buy vinyl sofas and vinyl chairs, fabric sofas and fabric chairs, or metal chairs?
Could we throw away any dead animal leather, suede, feathers, fur, or imitation fur, wool, animal prints, animal pictures products, of clothes and shoes and items?

Could we Stop doing this?

Could we stop eating, drinking, and wearing dead animals meat of: cow, chicken, egg, pig, fish, turkey, bee honey,
shrimp, crab, lobster, oyster, deer, turkey, goat, and other animals?

Could we stop drinking and eating alive and dead animal's products of milk, cheese, butter, sour cream, cottage cheese,
ice cream, yogurt, whey, ranch, and chocolate?

Could we stop using animal cow leather skins and cow suede of leather shoes, cow leather coats, cow leather vests,
cow leather pants, cow leather belts, cow leather wallets, cow leather purses, cow leather hats, cow leather car seats,
cow leather sofas, cow leather chairs, cow leather motorcycles, animal rugs, bird feather pillows, bird feather comforters,
bird eagle feather costumes, bird eagle feather hats, and bird feather earrings, bird feather coats, wool, animal prints and pictures?

Could we stop using so much of pots, stoves, ovens, microwaves, blenders, juicers, mixers, waffle machines, toasters,
toaster ovens, dehydrators, refrigerators, freezers, can openers, spiral slicers? And eat the foods whole. And use the counter
for our food where the sun light still shines on the fruit and vegetables, at room temperature, not so cold in the refrigerator.

At the Top of the Food World

Businesses of Gardens and Farms, of plants and trees, of how food should be for the people.
1. **"Farmers"** plant and pick, fruits and vegetables, and water, to feed the people of the citys, of the world.
2. **"Food Stores and Other Stores"** supply and sell the new foods, and cotton, linen, vinyl and fleece clothes and shoes.
3. **"Homes"** only purchase food from gardens and farms, from plants and trees, of fruits and vegetables, and water.

Businesses of Animals, that were made into food and items, and sold, to the people, how it should not be.
1. **Hunters of Land animals** – hunted alive and dead animals, and sold them for food and items, to the business of animals.
2. **Hunters of Air animals** – hunted alive and dead animals, and sold them for food and items to business of animals.
3. **Hunters of Ocean animals** – hunted alive and dead animals, and sold them, for food to business of animals.

4. **Business of Animals:** bought from hunters, death, and cut up animals, and made food of animal meat, and milk drinks of:

cows, chickens, pigs, fish, turkey, bee honey, shrimp, crab, lobster, crawfish, deer, sheep, goats, and other animals.

Business manufacture of cow or goat of milk and dairy items: of milk, cheese, butter, sour cream, cottage cheese,

ice cream, yogurt, whey, ranch, and chocolate.

Business manufacture of cow, birds, sheep, fox, rabbit: leather, fur, feathers, wool: shirts, pants, skirts, vests, coats, hats, gloves.

Business manufacture of cow, leather skins: shoes and boots.

Business manufacture of cow, leather skins: wallets, purses, bags and items accessories.

Business manufacture of cow, leather skins: sofas, chairs, rugs.

Business manufacture of cow, leather skins: car seats, and truck seats

Business manufacture of cow, leather skins: motorcycle seats and bags

Business manufacture of animals bodies: wall mounted animals, stuffed animals.

5. **Food Stores** - of animal meat and dairy milk drinks, and milk foods sold.
6. **Restaurants** - of animal meat and dairy milk drinks and milk foods sold.
7. **Fast Food Restaurants** - of animal meat and dairy milk drinks, and milk foods sold.
8. **Fuel Stations** - of animal meat and dairy milk drinks and milk foods sold.
9. **Convenient Stores** - of animal meat and dairy milk drinks, and milk foods sold.
10. **Work Office Buildings** - of animal meat and dairy milk drinks, and milk foods sold.
11. **Colleges and Schools** - serving animal meat and dairy milk drinks, and milk foods sold.
12. **"Homes Family"** – animal meat and dairy milk drinks and milk foods, start from here, to stop the animal foods bought and eaten, purchase fruit and vegetables, and water instead.
13. **"Individual Person"** - start here, to stop the eating, and drinking, of animals, of meat and dairy milk drinks. choose and decide, to eat only fresh foods, of fruits and vegetables, and drink water.

Could we stop following the crowd, of eating dead animal's milk and meat drinks and foods?
Be an individual of new foods alone, at home, and in the citys of the countries of the world around us, for the earth environment. Let's get back to the start of the world, where they ate only from the gardens and farms, not from the animals. Put farm fruit and vegetables in your body. Your body should be a garden and farm body filled with fruits and vegetables. Not a dead zoo body, filled with dead animals. We should have a body filled with fruits and vegetables with water only in our life, on earth now.

Here are some Positive Suggestions, for New Food People, of Fruits, Vegetables, and Water:

Could we eat garden and farm foods new, every day of our life, of fruits and vegetables, today, tomorrow, and forever?
Could we drink pure water fresh from the kitchen sink filtered, or bottled pour it into a glass so you don't have to drink words.
Could we make and wear cotton, linen, fleece, and vinyl, plain color materials and fabric, modest clothes, and shoes?

Could we plant a garden or farm, and fruit trees, in the back yard, or near an apartment, or on some city's land?

Could we take a walk each week, in the city, or at parks in nature, during the day or night?

Could we talk, and get to know each other as a couple, and spending time together, him and her?

Could we spend time alone, and get to know ourselves, more in the quiet?

Could we save money for a house, condo, or apartment?

Could we make and purchase furniture that is metal and wood, fabric, or plastic, not leather cow skins?

Could we make and drive in cars, trucks, motorcycles, that have fabric or vinyl seats only, not leather seats?

Could we purchase only what you need to have?

Could we have a nice business of work?

Could we pay our items on time, and stay out of debt?

Could we sleep early at night, to get a nice night of sleep, and wake up in the morning?

Could we wait for the one we are to be with, and date only them, and stay with them together, him and her?

Could you underline, what you ate and drank, and circle what you want to eat and drink?

Fruits

Grapefruit, Blue Berries, Black Berries, Raspberries, Cherries, Apple, Pear, Plum, Peach, Watermelon, Green Melon, Cantaloupe, Nectarine

Vegetables

Lettuce, Spinach, Basil, Red Tomato, Yellow Tomato, Broccoli, Cauliflower, Yellow Squash, Zucchini, Hiccima, Potato Brown,

Sweet Potatoe, Red Potatoe, Yellow Potato, Yam, Red Pepper, Green Pepper, Yellow Pepper, Carrots, Avocado, Asparagus, Lemon, Lime

Drinks

Water

Fruit Juice, Vegetable Juice, Soy Milk, Almond Milk, Tea Herbal

Energy Drinks, Clear Carbonated Drinks, Dark Carbonated Drinks, Alcohol, Coffee, Decaf Coffee, Milk of a Cow,

Lemonade, Tea Caffeine

Cooked Foods Vegetarian, no meat or dairy

Pizza no cheese, Spaghetti and sauce no meat, Bread, Bagels, Potato, Beans, Cereal and Soy Milk, Oatmeal, Grits, Hash Browns, Pancakes, Biscuits, Waffles, Noodles, Soups, Peanut Butter and Jell, Rice, Cooked Vegetables, Cooked Fruit in cans, Blended Fruit or Vegetables, Juiced Fruits, Juiced Vegetables, Veggie Burger and French Fries, Cinnamon Roll.

Dairy of Animals don't eat.

Cow Milk, Cow Cheese, Cow Butter, Cow Sour Cream, Cow Cottage Cheese, Cow Yogurt, Cow Ice Cream,

Cow Chocolate, Cow Whey, Cow Ranch

Meat of Animals don't eat or use.

Cow Meat, Cow Milk Products, Cow Leather

Chicken Meat, Chicken Eggs, Chicken Feather Pillows and Comforters

Pig Meat, Turkey Meat, Lamb Meat

Fish Meat, Shrimp Meat, Crab Meat, Lobster Tail Meat, Oysters and Pearls, Crawfish

Deer Meat, Deer Head Wall Placks

Goat Milk

Other Animals Heads Wall Placks

Bird Feathers Clothes and Hats

Bee Honey

All of these Animals should not be eaten.

Eat Fruit and Vegetables and drink water instead.

Could we eat and drink only New Garden and Farm Foods?
Could we do this for breakfast, lunch, dinner, and snacks?
Could we do this every day?

Food Plants and Food Trees, are from the Gardens and Farms, of the Land and Earth.

Food of new, fruit and vegetables, all sit still and quiet for months while they grow.

Food don't cook in a hot oven or on the stove, they are warmed and cooked, by the sun.

Food don't sit in the cold refrigerator all day, and in the cold dark refrigerator all night too.

Food sit on the ground on the gardens and farms, in the sunlight all day, and the cool of the night.

Food grow from the trees high in the air.

Food grow in plants above the ground.

They grow on the ground on the soil.

They grow under the ground in the soil.

Food don't move around.

Food drink only water, rain.

Food don't eat animal's bodies, or animal's fluids of dairy milk .

Food wear mostly only one color all their life.

Food are all plants for us to eat, and be like them.

Food of new, fruit and vegetables, are all filled with pure water, air, sunshine and moon light.

Food has many colors of the rainbow for us to eat.

Food are there for us to eat for breakfast, lunch, dinner, and snacks new.

Foods from the gardens and farms, of plants and trees, from A to Z, of fruits and vegetables. Could you eat all of them.

A   apple, avocado, almond, argula, alfalfa sprouts, artichoke

B   banana, blueberry, blackberry, broccoli, brussel sprout, basil, bok choy, all beans

C   carrot, cherry, cantaloupe, cauliflower, cabbage, celery, coconut white, coconut brown, cilantro, cashew, currants, cranberries
D   durian
E   egg plant – could we call that black plant, endive, endamame
F   fig
G   grape, grapefruit, green beans
H   honeydew melon
I   iceberg lettuce
J   jicama, jalapeno
K   kale
L   lettuce, lime
M   mushroom
N   nectarine
O   orange, black olive
P   pear, peach, plum, potato, pepper, parsley, papaya, pecan, peanut, peas, pineapple
Q   quince
R   radish, raspberry, rhubarb, rice
S   spinach, sweet potato, squash, starfruit
T   tomato, tangerine
U   uzouza leaf
V   vanilla
W   watermelon, walnut, wheat, water
X   xigua
Y   yam, yuzu, yellow squash
Z   zucchini

When eating cut out the seeds and spoon them out.
Could you not eat the seeds of all the fruits and vegetables?
I cut and spoon out the seeds in the tomato and banana.
Fruits, vegetables and nuts are the healthiest for us we, new.
We are thankful for them, to feed us daily in our life A to Z.

Could We Stop Drinking & Eating Animals?

cows, chickens, pigs, turkeys, fishes, shrimps, crabs, lobsters, crawfishes, deers, bees honey, eggs, lambs, oysters, other animals

milk – from a cow or goat
butter or margarine - from a cow
cheese - from a cow
sour cream - from a cow
cottage cheese - from a cow
yogurt - from a cow
ice cream – from a cow

chocolate – from a cow
whey – from a cow
ranch– from a cow
egg – from a chicken
mayonnaise – egg in it - from a chicken
chicken – body parts or all
cow - meat, steak, hamburger, beef
turkey – from a bird
pig - bacon, rib, pork roast, sausage,
hot dog, bologna, pork chips, ham
fish – fish sticks, fish, salmon, halibit
shrimp, crawfish, crab, lobster
lamb – from a sheep
bee honey – from an insect
other animals

Could we not use Electric Kitchen Cooking Machines?

ovens, pots on stoves, microwaves, juicers, blenders, food processors, spiral slicer, dehydrator, waffle machine, refrigerator, freezer, can opener, mixers,
coffee machine, tea machine, toaster, toaster oven, crock pot, and other machines.

Its best to not cook food, and could you eat them new?

Could We Stop Using Animal Leather, Suede, Fur,
Fake Fur, Feathers, Wool, and Animal Fabric Prints?

cow skin leather and suede – shirts, vests, pants, skirts, coats, hats, gloves
cow skin leather and suede – shoes, boots
cow skin leather - purses, wallets, jewelry, other items
cow skin leather – sofas, chairs, and fur rugs
cow skin leather - cars, truck, motorcycle, seats
animal fur and imitation fur – coats, pillows, blankets, rugs
bird feathers - coats, hats, jewelry, other items
wool sheep – clothes, shirts, suits
animal fabric material prints -clothes, other items

Could we ware cotton, linen, fleece, velvet, and vinyl fabrics?
Could We Eat All New Garden and Farm Foods?

Fruit
Apple
Grapefruit

Grape
Peach
Plum
Banana
Orange
Blackberry
Blueberry
Pineapple
Raspberry
Cherry
Cantaloupe
Watermelon
Coconut

Vegetables
Lettuce, Spinach
Potato, Sweet Potato
Zucchini
Red Pepper, Green Pepper, Yellow Pepper
Tomato Red, Tomato Yellow
Yellow squash
Carrot
Cauliflower
Avocado
Black Olive
Rice, Wheat

Nuts – new, not roasted or salted
Almond, Peanuts, Cashews, Pecans, Walnuts, Macadamia

Water - from the kitchen sink filtered, or bottled,
pour the water into a glass, so you don't have to drink words.

Could we plant a garden or farm, of fruit and vegetables,
fruit trees, nut trees, and plants that make food of the land and earth?

Could we keep the foods on the counter, like on a farm,
at Nature's temperature, instead the cold refrigerator and freezer?

Could we cut out the seeds, from the foods of fruits and vegetables?
Could we not eat the seeds of the foods?

We could cut out the seeds, out of bananas and tomatos, and other foods,
and not eat the seeds, eat the fruit and vegetables seedless.

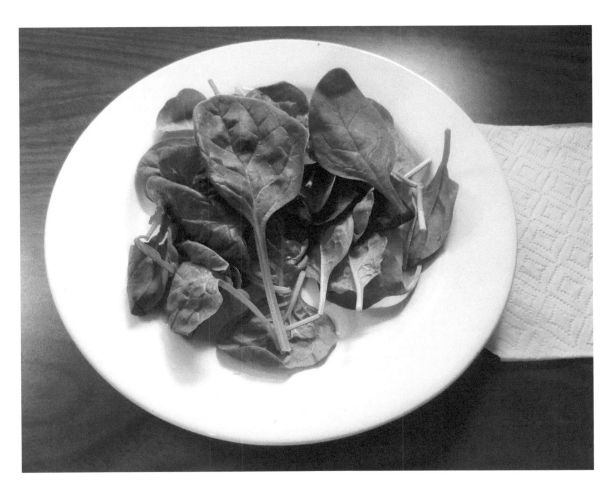

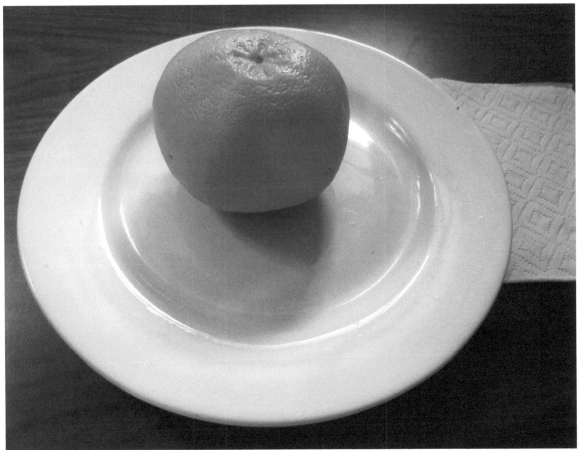

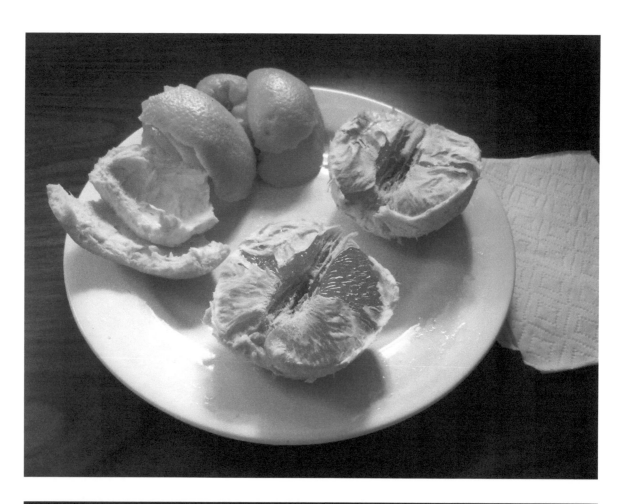

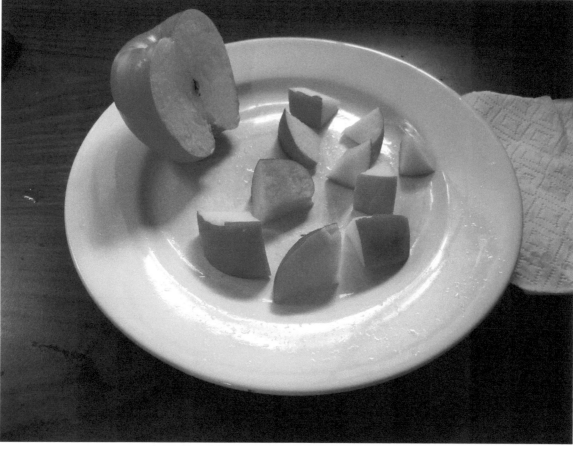

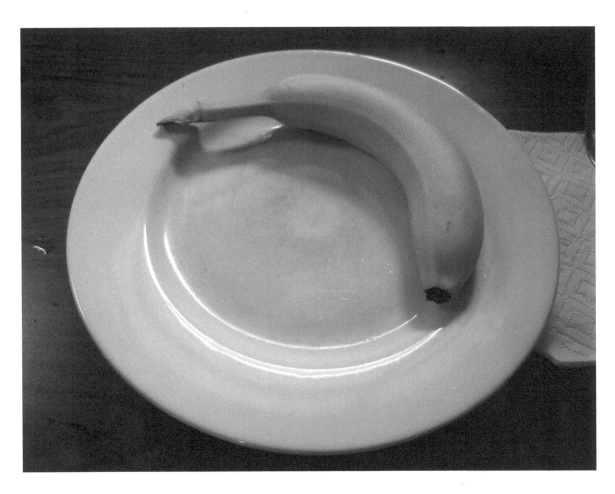

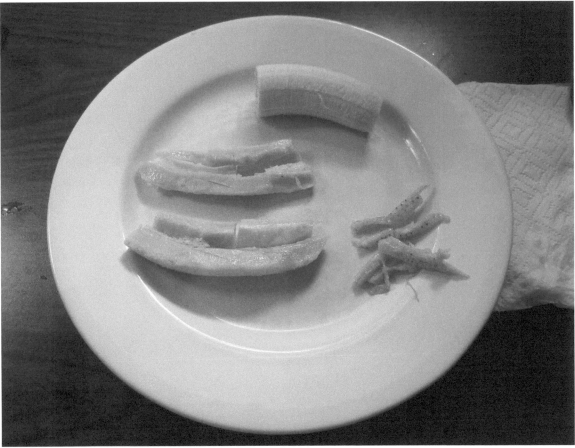

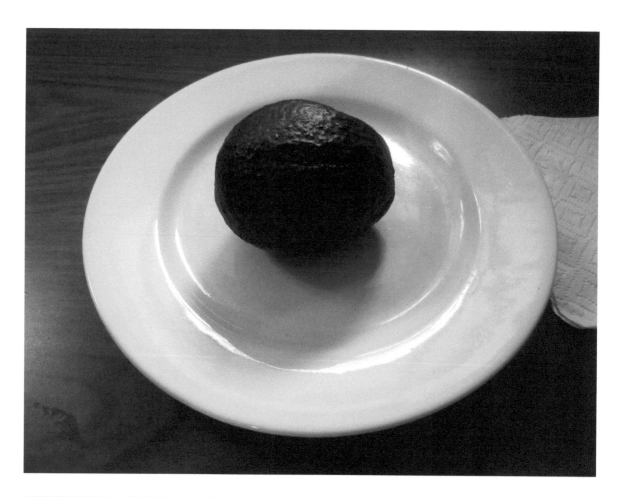

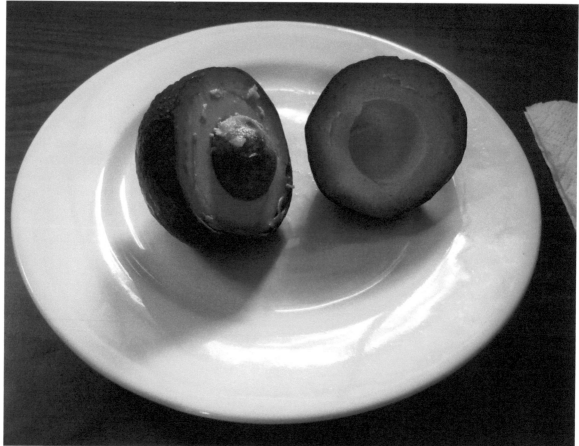

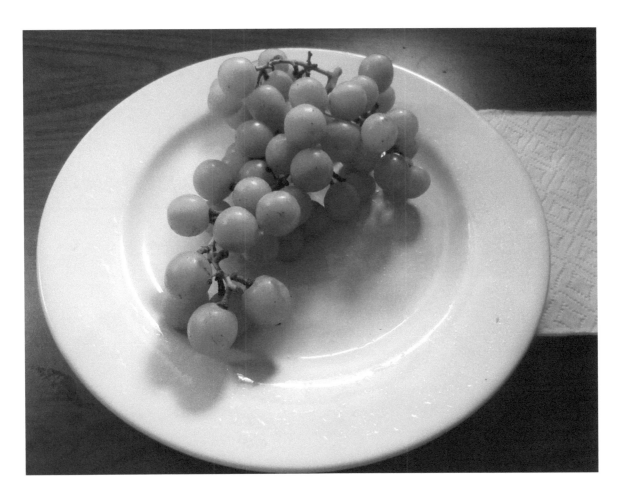

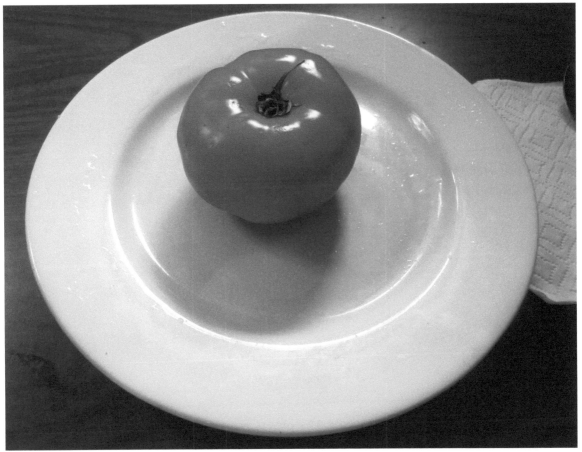

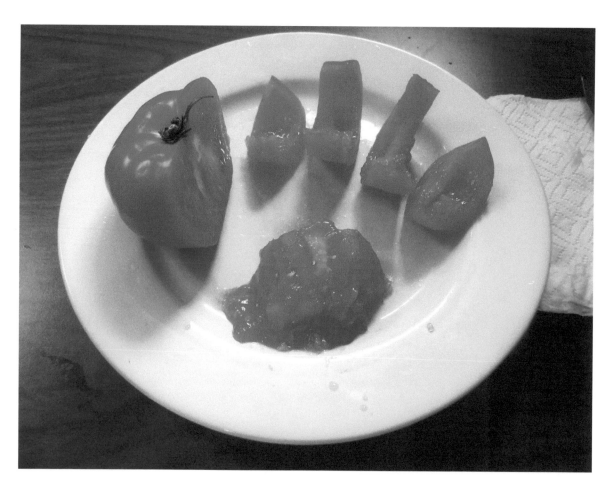

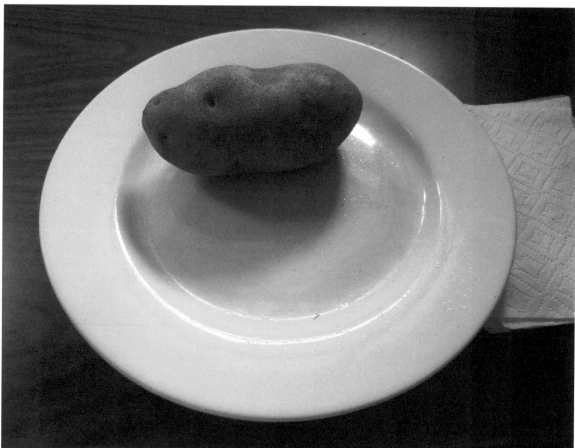

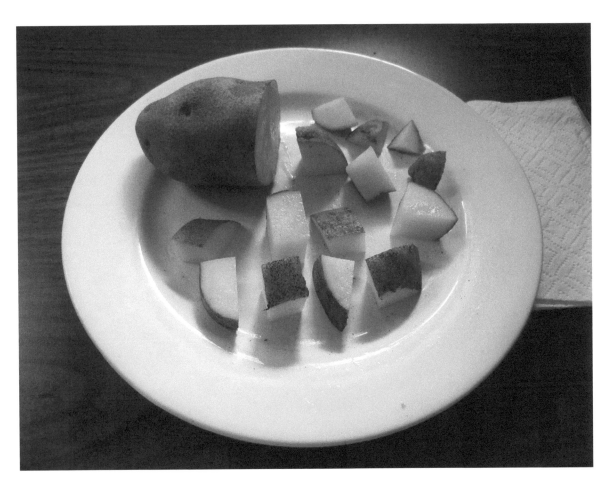

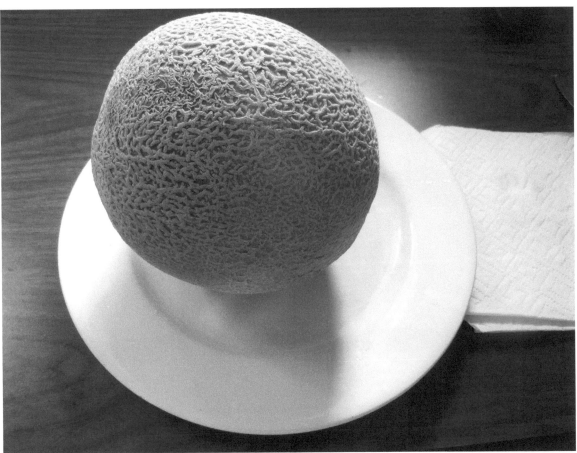

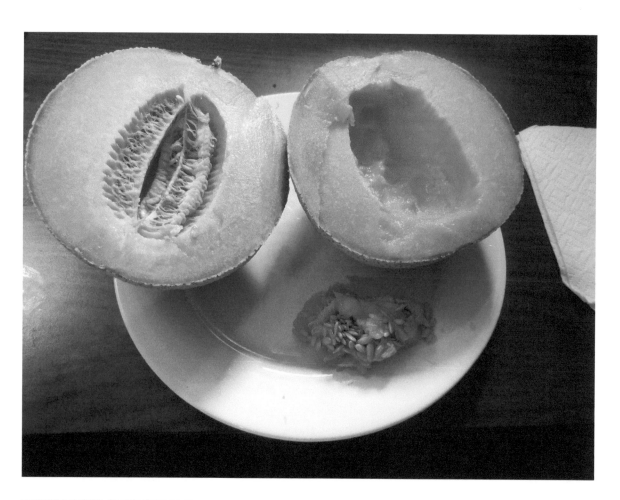

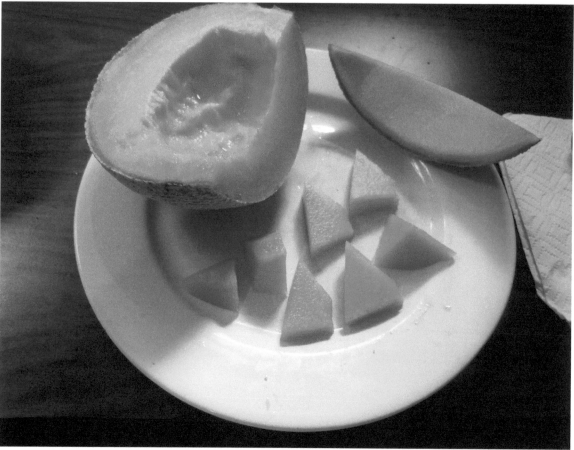

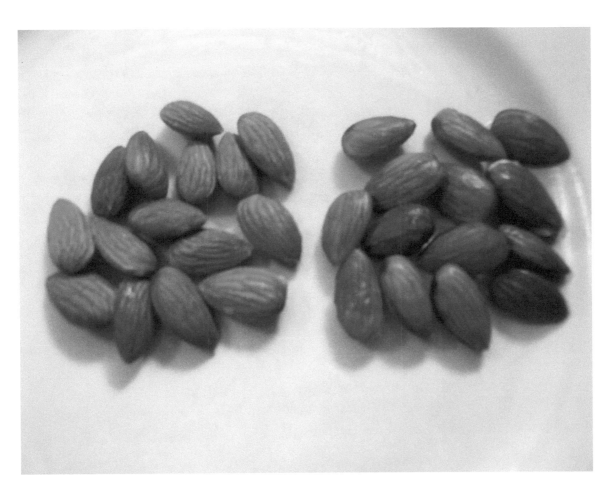

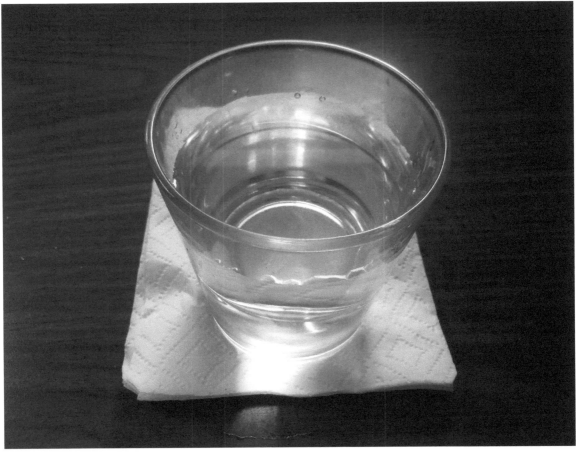